1984

HOSPITAL PURCHASING

Focus on Effectiveness

Editor
Charles E. Housley
Saint Anthony Hospital
Columbus, Ohio

A collection of articles from *Hospital Materiel Management Quarterly*

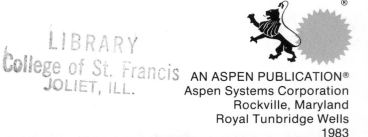

AN ASPEN PUBLICATION®
Aspen Systems Corporation
Rockville, Maryland
Royal Tunbridge Wells
1983

Library of Congress Cataloging in Publication Data
Main entry under title:

Hospital purchasing

"A collection of articles from Hospital materiel
management quarterly."
Includes index.
1. Hospitals—Purchasing—Addresses, essays, lectures.
I. Housley, Charles E. II. Hospital materiel management
quarterly. [DNLM: 1. Purchasing, Hospital—Collected
works. 2. Materiels Management, Hospital—Economics—
Collected works. WX 157 H831]
RA 971.33.H665   1983   362.1'1'0687   83-11793
ISBN 0-89443-819-0

Publisher: John Marozsan
Editor in Chief: Michael Brown
Publications Editor: Kenneth E. Lawrence
Executive Managing Editor: Margot Raphael
Printing and Manufacturing: Nina Kasari

Library of Congress Catalog Card Number: 83-11793
ISBN: 0-89443-819-0

Printed in the United States of America

1   2   3   4   5

Contents

Introduction

Purchasing has always intrigued hospital materiel managers, and recently negotiation has also come into the limelight. There is a distinct difference between these two materiel functions. By definition, negotiation is the process by which a materiel manager arranges for and brings about terms, conditions, and quality of purchase through enlightened discussion, conference, and compromise. Purchasing is the simple act of drawing from the terms of results-oriented negotiation. Negotiation should always precede purchasing, and for best results, the two should never be combined into the same function.

There are several reasons for the upsurge of interest in purchasing and negotiation. The primary reason for the hospital's views of purchasing's importance is the fact that this function takes up an entire department. Purchasing and negotiation receive attention because regulatory bodies and third party intermediaries have placed great emphasis on hospital cost containment and purchasing power. Government Accounting Office (GAO) studies, for example, have created turmoil in the purchasing field; Blue Cross is promoting interest in price sharing and price systems; and the American Hospital Association, as well as the individual state associations, places a great deal of emphasis on cost containment. The emphasis of these intermediaries affects the thought process of hospital administrators, materiel managers, and purchasing directors.

Another reason for the interest is that the results of purchasing and negotiation, and therefore the efficiency of these functions are quantifiably measurable. Many of the functions of materiel management are not measurable in terms of dollars and cents, but purchasing is. As long as it is felt that measuring the effectiveness of purchasing is important, there will be some group—hospitals, third party payers, or government regulatory bodies—in search of that elusive "best price."

Purchasing is also receiving a great deal of administrative attention because it and some of its corollaries, such as inventory control, are prime areas for automation. Industry has done a tremendous amount of data gathering and retrieval in the area of purchasing by using computers. Hospitals see purchasing as a prime target for the use of data processing, information systems.

In this day of computers and advanced technology, it is easy to lose sight of some basic principles of materiel management. Today's trend seems to be that systems must be complex to be worth considering—they must be computerized, centralized, pressurized, automated, integrated, or amalgamated to get managers' attention. It is a sobering thought that all materiel management systems are based on purchasing and negotiation.

Simplicity is beautiful. In hospitals that are having problems in materiel management, often the most basic principles have been violated. If a hospital is having problems with its perpetual inventory system, computerizing its inventory will not solve the problems. Computers will not correct human or management errors. Good supervision will; machines cannot. As has often been said of computers, if garbage goes in, garbage will come out (GIGO).

Hospitals are facing double-digit inflation, unbalanced budgets, uncontrollable costs, and insistence on cost containment by third parties and government. What an atmosphere in which to discuss reducing and containing costs! However, there is room for most hospitals "to tighten their belts," and one of the most promising areas to begin with is that of materiel costs. This is primarily why purchasing and negotiation have gained so much attention recently. Hospital purchasing directors in the past shopped for quality, price, and service, in that order; but times have changed. Today quality is almost taken for granted because so many agencies are monitoring the packaging, sterilizing, storage, and distribution of supplies. Reputable companies are expected to maintain high quality control standards for their name-brand items. Price is still a negotiable term, but it too has lost some of its appeal with the hospital's thrust toward purchasing in large dollar volumes through prime suppliers, group purchasing, and shared service endeavors. Hospitals must put their emphasis on bargaining and negotiate for service in the supply sector now and in the future. After all, what good are excellent quality and price if the item cannot be obtained?

Purchasing, not to be confused with nego-tiation, is probably one of the least important materiel functions. Materiel distribution, supply, process, and distribution and the general materiel flow within the hospital are more important than the act of purchasing. Certainly, this is proved when the total function of materiel management is examined. In many hospitals, the hospital purchasing director can save twice the price normally paid and still come out financially ahead if the materiel is managed and used effectively within the institution. However, as long as purchasing remains important to the hospitals, third party payers, and government regulatory bodies, purchasing will continue to receive the bulk of the attention.

In this book, I have particularly and justifiably dealt with the fundamental and advanced stages of purchasing and negotiation. I have selected authors and articles that represent some of the best thinking on the subject of purchasing and negotiation, such as: S. Randolph Hayas's article entitled "Total Centralized Purchasing: Can It Ever Be Achieved?" and Diane M. Signoracci's article on "Effective Hospital Purchasing." Attorney Michael K. Gire has well represented the legal aspects of purchasing in his articles, "Avoiding Conflict of Interest and Related Organization Problems" and "Hospital Procurement and Illegal Price Discrimination." The advanced stages of purchasing are addressed in the articles by William H. Rosegay, "Computerized Purchasing, Materiel Management and Accounts Payable Systems: Planning, Features and Selection," and by William H. Henning's "Utilizing Suppliers to the Hospital's Best Interests." Purchasing and negotiation of capital equipment are also capably dealt with in the following articles: Charles C. Crider's "Capital Equipment Acquisition," Steven R. Campbell's "Procurement of Major Equipment," George P. Page's "A Comparative Analysis of a Cost-Plus Purchasing System and a Pricing Service Program," and Elbert O. Garner's

"Hospital Capital Equipment Purchasing in an Investor-Owned Environment."

This book also represents the best present-day thinking on group purchasing as depicted by the following articles: David M. Baker's "Group Purchasing—The Great Debate," Charles E. Housley's "Overcoming Barriers to Group Purchasing," Craig W. Moore's "Group Purchasing: Past, Present and Future," Oren M. Williams, Jr.'s "Group Purchasing: A Vendor's Perspective," Richard S. Lovering's "Minimizing the Antitrust Risks of Group Purchasing,"

and Richard L. Sim's "Group Purchasing Makes Sense: An Administrator's Perspective." These are but a few of the excellent articles included in this anthology of purchasing literary works.

I am sure you will find this book interesting, informative, and a source of motivation in providing hospitals with the best possible leadership in this very important arena.

Charles E. Housley
August 1983

Effective hospital purchasing

Diane M. Signoracci
Associate
Bricker & Eckler
Columbus, Ohio

A PURCHASE ORDER is typically a written form document, drawn up by the prospective buyer of goods and sent by that buyer to a prospective seller of the goods. A written purchase order is preferred to an oral order because the writing memorializes the substance of the agreement sought by the buyer. It protects the buyer from unbargained-for terms in the event of misunderstandings and disputes under that agreement. The typed or written information on the purchase order describes the goods and specific terms of the bargain sought by the buyer on that particular purchase; the printed information sets forth the general terms sought by the buyer on all of its standard purchases.

In legal terms a purchase order often represents the buyer's "offer" to purchase goods from the seller, giving the seller the power of "acceptance." If the seller accepts the offer by either sending the buyer a confirming acknowledgment or by shipping goods that conform to the buyer's offer, then a contract is formed. Therefore, because a purchase order may ripen into a contract upon its acceptance by the seller, it is important that it be complete in all contract terms.

The face of the purchase order should provide the specific information relevant to the purchase. Such information should include the name and address of the seller and the buyer, description of the merchandise, shipping instructions, delivery terms, and payment terms. A sample face sheet of a hospital purchase order and the general terms and conditions that appear on its reverse side are presented in the Appendix.

The sample purchase order in the appendix contains terms and conditions favorable to the hospital-buyer. Consequently it is not unlikely that, on receipt of such a probuyer purchase order, a hospital supplier would either ship the goods ordered or acknowledge the purchase order without adopting the prohospital terms of that order. Instead, the supplier's documents are likely to contain terms and conditions favorable to the seller, and one of those terms may provide, as did the hospital's purchase order, that the supplier's invoice or acknowledgment is the complete and final agreement between the parties. Given the likelihood of competing forms, questions arise as to (1) which form will control transactions under the purchase agreement and (2) how the hospital can draft a purchase order to guarantee that its terms and not the terms of its supplier will control the purchase agreement.

HISTORICAL PERSPECTIVE

Common law approach

In common law, before adoption of the Uniform Commercial Code, any response to the hospital's offer to purchase goods, other than a "mirror image" of that offer (accepting all terms and conditions), would not have constituted acceptance of the hospital's offer. A supplier's invoice or acknowledgment that contained terms different from or in addition to the hospital's terms would have represented a counteroffer by the supplier to the hospital, which the hospital would have been free either to accept or reject. If the hospital, however, accepted the goods (even without expressly accepting the supplier's terms), the hospital would have been deemed to have accepted the goods subject to the terms of the supplier's "counteroffer."

The common law approach to competing forms presented significant problems. The time of contract formation was unrealistic. By delaying contract formation until the buyer's acceptance of the seller's counteroffer, the common law allowed the buyer to back out of the agreement for reasons other than conflicting contract terms—e.g., lower prices elsewhere. However, if the buyer accepted the goods, the common law approach was significantly proseller, imposing the terms of the seller on the buyer.

Code approach

The official text of the code was promulgated in 1951. It provided a body of law that governs commercial transactions. Although not enacted by the U.S. Congress as a general statutory law, the code has been enacted by 49 states (Louisiana being the exception), the District of Columbia, and the Virgin Islands. Because the code is enacted locally, some variations among the jurisdictions may occur as to exact wording; therefore it is important when working with the code to consult the local codification.

The code replaces any number of often-conflicting state statutes in the area of commercial transactions, including the Uniform Sales Act, the Negotiable Instruments Law, a number of so-called "uniform" acts concerned with bills of lading, warehouse receipts, conditional sales, and statutes dealing with the financing of commercial transactions. Hospital purchases of goods would be governed by Article 2 of the code, which deals with transactions in goods.

COMPETING FORMS

The drafters of the code attempted to resolve the problems of the common law approach to competing forms in Section 2-207, which reads in full:

(1) A definite and reasonable expression of acceptance or a written confirmation which is sent within a reasonable time operates as an acceptance even though it states terms additional to or different from those offered or agreed upon, unless acceptance is expressly made conditional on assent to the additional or different terms.
(2) The additional terms are to be construed as proposals for addition to the contract. Between merchants such terms become part of the contract unless:

  (a) the offer expressly limits acceptance to the terms of the offer;
  (b) they materially alter it; or
  (c) notification of objection to them has already been given or is given within a reasonable time after notice of them is received.

(3) Conduct by both parties which recognizes

the existence of a contract is sufficient to establish a contract for sale although the writings of the parties do not otherwise establish a contract. In such case the terms of the particular contract consist of those terms on which the writings of the parties agree, together with any supplementary terms incorporated under any other provision of this Act.

Section 2-207 cuts into the common law mirror image or counteroffer approach to competing forms. It provides for contract formation on the exchange of forms, regardless of the presence of competing terms. Between nonmerchants the terms of the buyer's offer become the terms of the contract, and the additional terms of the seller become proposals for additions to the contract, which require the buyer's assent for inclusion in the contract.

Between merchants, such additional terms automatically become part of the contract unless: the offer expressly limits acceptance to its terms; the additional terms materially alter the contract; or the buyer objects to the terms within a reasonable time. The operation and purpose of Section 2-207 may become confused when either or both parties include a clause within their respective documents that insists on all its terms for contract formation.

HYPOTHETICAL CASE

As relevant to hospital purchases, the operation of Section 2-207 can best be explained by the use of a hypothetical situation. Assume that the hospital offers to purchase goods from the hospital supplier. The hospital's purchase order provides for a warranty that the goods purchased will be free from defects; the purchase order is silent on arbitration. Assume that the supplier responds with an acknowledgment that disclaims any warranty for the quality of the goods and provides that all disputes under the contract will be submitted for arbitration. The supplier ships the goods, which the hospital accepts and pays for. Assume further that a dispute concerning the quality of the goods arises. Does a contract exist between the hospital and the supplier? If so, which terms under the contract are controlling?

If the dickered terms—for example, price, quantity, description of goods, delivery terms, and payment terms— appearing on the face of the hospital's purchase order and the seller's acknowledgment agree, then a contract is formed on exchange of these documents. If the dickered terms, however, do not agree, no contract is formed under Section 2-207(1), because the supplier's acknowledgment would not be a "definite and reasonable expression of acceptance" of the hospital's offer. Generally the typed or written terms of the printed form documents must agree for contract formation on exchange of forms. For purposes of this hypothetical situation, assume that the dickered terms agree.

DISCLAIMERS AND ADDITIONS

Under Section 2-207, regardless of the competing terms, the supplier's acknowledgment represents an acceptance of the hospital's offer, at which time a contract is formed on the hospital's terms. But what about the supplier's disclaimer and arbitration provisions? Section 2-207(2) provides that "additional" terms are to be construed

as proposals for addition to the contract. However only the supplier's arbitration provision literally represents an "additional" term, because the hospital's purchase order was silent on this point. The supplier's disclaimer is not an "additional" term but a "different" term, because it conflicts with the hospital's warranty provision. Although Section 2-207(1) permits contract formation in the presence of both "additional" and "different" terms, Section 2-207(2) provides that only "additional" terms are to be construed as proposals for addition to the contract.

Interpretations

The use of the words "different" and "additional" in Section 2-207(1) and the use of only the word "additional" in subsection 2 have given rise to a variety of interpretations from the courts and commentators. One view is that only additional terms will be considered as proposals for addition to the contract and that different terms will be excised from the agreement. The rationale of this approach is that subsection 2 literally applies to only "additional" terms and that the offerer cannot be expected to assent to conflicting terms.[1] In the hypothetical situation, under this approach, the supplier's disclaimer provision would be dropped from the agreement, and the hospital's warranty provision would control future negotiations and actions under the contract.

Another approach to the different-additional dichotomy is that the different terms will be cancelled out. The contract then consists of terms on which the parties are in agreement, and standard code provisions replace the conflicting terms.[2,3] The supporters of this approach emphasize the language of comment 6 to Section 2-207, which reads in part:

Where clauses on confirming forms sent by both parties conflict each party must be assumed to object to a clause of the other. . . . As a result the requirement that there be notice of objection which is found in subsection (2) is satisfied and the conflicting terms do not become part of the contract. The contract then consists of the terms originally expressly agreed to, terms on which the confirmations agree, and terms supplied by [the Code], including subsection (2).

Under this theory the hospital's warranty provision and the supplier's disclaimer clause would cancel out, and the code's implied warranties of merchantability and fitness for a particular purpose would control.

Some courts and commentators urge that subsection 2 is appropriately applied to different terms as well as additional terms, pointing to the language of comment 3 as support for their position.[4] Comment 3 to Section 2-207 provides that "[w]hether or not additional *or different* terms will become part of the agreement depends upon the provision of subsection (2). . . ." If this approach is adopted, the fate of the supplier's disclaimer provision as well as its arbitration provision will be determined under subsection 2.

Merchants' clause

Under subsection 2 of Section 2-207, the supplier's disclaimer provision and arbitration provision may automatically become additions to the contract, if the hospital and its supplier are considered to be "merchants." The code defines "merchant" in Section 2-104(1) as: "a person who deals in goods of the kind or otherwise by his occupation holds himself out as having knowledge or skill peculiar to the practices or goods involved in the transaction."

Comment 2 to Section 2-104 further states that:

Section [ ] . . . 2-207 . . . dealing with . . . confirmatory memoranda . . . rest[s] on normal business practices which are or ought to be typical of and familiar to any person in business. For purposes of [Section 2-207] almost every person in business would, therefore, be deemed to be a "merchant" under the language "when . . . by his occupation holds himself out as having knowledge or skill peculiar to the practices . . . involved in the transaction . . ." since the practices involved in the transaction are non-specialized business practices such as answering mail.

Given the language of the code and its comment, hospitals and their suppliers would be considered merchants for purposes of Section 2-207. Therefore, in the hypothetical situation, unless one of the three exceptions to subsection 2 applies, the supplier's disclaimer and arbitration clauses would become part of the contract.

Exceptions

Expressed limits

The first exception to the general rule of subsection 2 is found in paragraph a, which bars additional terms from becoming part of the bargain if "the offer expressly limits acceptance to the terms of the offer." If the hospital's purchase order expressly limits acceptance of the purchase order to the terms of that order, then the supplier's disclaimer and arbitration clauses would not become additions to the contract under subsection 2.

Materiality

Paragraph b, subsection 2, excludes additional terms that "materially alter" the contract from becoming part of that contract. Although the code does not define "material," comment 4 to Section 2-207 lists examples of typical clauses that would materially alter a contract. Among these examples is a clause negating standard warranties. Therefore under section 2-207(2)(b), the supplier's disclaimer provision would not become part of the contract, because it would be considered to materially alter the contract.

Neither the code nor its comments indicates whether the addition of an arbitration clause would be considered a material alteration of the contract. Some courts have held that an arbitration clause in a

---

Some courts have held that an arbitration clause in a seller's form is not a material alteration; other courts have reached the opposite conclusion.

---

seller's form is not a material alteration[5]; other courts have reached the opposite conclusion.[6,7] One court noted that whether or not an arbitration clause constitutes a material alteration within Section 2-207 is a question of fact to be determined in light of the circumstances of each particular case.[8]

Prior custom within an industry and course of dealing between parties are also considered in deciding this issue.[9,10] Therefore whether the supplier's arbitration clause would be excluded from the contract as a material alteration under Section 2-207(2)(b) might depend on the jurisdiction in which the action is brought, the circumstances of the transaction, the arbitration custom in the hospital supply industry, and previous dealings between the hospital and supplier.

Reasonable notification

Paragraph c of subsection 2 excludes additional terms from the contract when "notification of objection to them has already been given or is given within a reasonable time after notice of them is received." Because paragraph c allows for objection before the fact, the hospital could guarantee exclusion of the supplier's disclaimer and arbitration provisions by a clause in its purchase order that provides that "Buyer objects to any terms in addition to or different from the terms of this order."

If the foregoing clause is omitted from the purchase order, the hospital may still bar the disclaimer and arbitration provisions by notifying the supplier of the hospital's objection to those provisions. This notification, however, must be given within a reasonable time after the supplier's document containing the objectionable terms is delivered to the hospital or after such terms otherwise come to the attention of the hospital.[11] Code Section 1-204(2) provides that "a reasonable time for taking any action depends on the nature, purpose and circumstances of such action." However the provision of notice within a reasonable time does not require immediate action, and what is a reasonable time is ordinarily a question of fact.[12]

As with the question of materiality, the hospital must look at the surrounding circumstances, the custom within the hospital supply industry, and its prior dealings with this supplier to determine what is notice of objection within a "reasonable time." It is in the hospital's best interests to notify the supplier of its objection to the disclaimer and to arbitration provisions as promptly as possible.

HYPOTHETICAL COMPLICATION

To the proposed hypothetical situation add the assumption that either the hospital's purchase order or the supplier's acknowledgment contains a provision that insists on acceptance of or assent to all its terms and only its terms. The addition of such provision throws the agreement into analysis under the "expressly conditional" clause of subsection 1 of Section 2-207, which states in part that: "A definite and reasonable expression of acceptance . . . operates as an acceptance even though it states terms additional to or different from those offered . . . *unless acceptance is expressly made conditional on assent to the additional or different terms.*" The "expressly conditional" clause of subsection 1 precludes contract formation on the exchange of documents with conflicting or additional terms in which the documents of at least one party expressly insist on assent to or acceptance of all of its terms.

If the hospital's purchase order states: "This order can be accepted only by a document that consists of all the terms of this order and contains neither additional nor different terms," a contract under Section 2-207(1) would be formed only if the terms of the supplier's acknowledgment "mirrored" the buyer's terms. In the hypothetical situation no contract would

be formed because the supplier adds an arbitration provision and disclaims the warranties provided by the hospital's purchase order.

If the supplier's acknowledgment provides that: "Seller's acceptance is expressly conditioned on buyer's assent to the additional or different terms and conditions set forth herein," a contract would be formed on the exchange of documents only if the hospital assented to the supplier's disclaimer and arbitration provisions. It is reasonable to assume that the hospital would not assent to such provisions, and no contract would be formed.

Because no contract has been formed on the exchange of documents in the aforementioned situations, both the hospital and supplier would be free to back out of the agreement. However if each party chooses to perform under the agreement (i.e., if the supplier ships the goods ordered, and the hospital accepts and pays for such goods) a contract would be formed. The issue would remain, however, as to what terms govern future actions under the contract. Assume, as before, a dispute develops over the quality of the goods. The hospital claims breach of the purchase order's warranty provision and seeks standard judicial remedies. The supplier contends all warranties are disclaimed by its acknowledgment and that disputes are to be settled by arbitration.

COURT CASES

The courts on various occasions have addressed actual patterns similar to those of this hypothetical situation. In *Roto-Lith Ltd. v. F. P. Bartlett & Co.,*[13] the First

Circuit Court of Appeals addressed a situation in which the seller's acknowledgment contained a disclaimer that conflicted with the buyer's warranty provision, and in which the seller's acknowledgment was "expressly conditioned" on assent to all its terms.

Reverting to the common law approach, the court held that the seller's acknowledgment was not an acceptance of the buyer's offer but, instead, was a counteroffer to the buyer, which was accepted by the buyer upon its receipt and use of the goods. Because the buyer was held to have accepted the seller's counteroffer on the seller's terms, the seller in *Roto-Lith v. Bartlett* was given the benefit of its disclaimer. If this approach were adopted in the hypothetical situation, the supplier's acknowledgment would be characterized as a counteroffer. The hospital's acceptance of the goods ordered would be deemed an acceptance of the supplier's counteroffer and an assent to the counteroffer's terms, including disclaimer and arbitration provisions.

The common law approach to competing forms with "expressly conditional" clauses, as adopted by the *Roto-Lith v. Bartlett* decision, has been subjected to severe criticism by commentators.[14] More importantly the approach has not been followed in numerous decisions involving the battle of the forms under Section 2-207.[15-18]

The decision of the Seventh Circuit Court in *C. Itoh & Co. v. Jordan International Co.* represents the more widely accepted approach to cases involving competing forms with "expressly conditional" clauses.[19] The court found that no contract arose on exchange of documents by virtue of Section 2-207(1) because the seller had conditioned acceptance on the buyer's consent to an arbitration clause. The Seventh Circuit Court rejected the *Roto-Lith v. Bartlett* decision, however, and refused to find the buyer's acceptance of the goods tantamount to acceptance of the seller's counteroffer. The court based its opinion on the language of Section 2-207(3), which reads:

Conduct by both parties which recognizes the existence of a contract is sufficient to establish a contract for sale although the writings ... do not.... In such case the terms of the particular contract consist of those terms on which the writings of the parties agree, together with any supplementary terms incorporated under any other provisions of [the Code].

The court found that under subsection 3 a contract arose when both parties proceeded with performance as though there were a contract. However the court, quoting subsection 3, held that the contract did not include the additional terms of the seller but was limited to "those terms in which the writings of the parties agreed, together with any supplementary terms incorporated under any other provision of [the Code]."[20]

SELLER DISADVANTAGE

It is important to note that contract formation under Section 2-207(3) gives neither the buyer nor the seller the disputed terms in its document; subsection 3 instead fills out the contract with standardized provisions of the code. As a practical matter, however, contract formation under Section 2-207(3) may put the seller at a disadvantage, because the seller will often wish to undertake less responsibility for the quality of its goods than the standard provisions of the code impose.

In the hypothetical situation posed, contract formation under Section 2-207(3) would result in the excision of the supplier's arbitration provision. Because the code does not provide for standard arbitration terms, no code provision would replace the excised term, and disputes under the hypothetical contract would not be subject to arbitration. Furthermore both the hospital's warranty and the supplier's disclaimer would drop out of the agreement and be replaced by the implied warranty provisions of the code.

Hospital management can use the code to provide the hospital with a more favorable purchasing agreement than was available under common law. Hospital management, however, must structure its purchasing procedure to take full advantage of code provisions. All purchases should be documented by a written purchase order. The purchase order itself should consist of terms that are favorable as well as necessary to the hospital's interests as the buyer of goods. Hospital management, however, should not expect that in every purchase the supplier will agree to all the terms of the hospital's purchase order; and management should anticipate a prosupplier form document in response to its probuyer purchase order.

CRITICAL LANGUAGE

Section 2-207's approach to the battle of the forms is more favorable to the buyer. However there is probably no language that can be inserted in a purchase order that will guarantee the hospital—as purchaser—of forming a contract on its terms, if the hospital's supplier responds to that purchase order with a form acknowledgment that requires assent to all of the supplier's terms. Language can be inserted, however, that will assure the hospital of not forming a contract on the supplier's terms, that language being: "the buyer objects to any terms in addition to or different from the terms of this order."

This language, while protecting the hospital from unfavorable terms of the supplier, may result in contract formation under subsection 3, in which case neither party will receive the disputed terms of its forms. Still, under Section 2-207(3), the standard code provisions, that replace the cancelled competing terms of the buyer's and seller's forms, are often more likely to favor the hospital as offerer. If, however, the hospital demands a particular term, the hospital should try to make such term a "written in" or "dickered" term of the agreement. If the supplier refuses to negotiate on the term, the hospital may have to decide whether it is more advantageous to forget the entire agreement or to live without the disputed term.[21]

REFERENCES

1. Air Products & Chemical, Inc. v. Fairbanks, Morse, Inc., 58 Wis. 2d 193, 206 N.W. 2d 414 (1973).
2. Idaho Pipe & Steel Co. v. Cal-Cut Pipe & Supply, Inc., 98 Idaho 495, 567 P. 2d 1246 (1977).
3. Lea Tai Textile Co. v. Manning Fabrics, Inc., 411 F. Supp. 1404 (S. D. N. Y. 1975).
4. Ebasco Services, Inc. v. Pennsylvania Power & Light Co., 402 F. Supp. 421 (E. D. Pa. 1975).

5. Gaynor-Stafford Industries, Inc. v. Mafco Textured Fibers, 52 A.D.2d 481, 384 N.Y.S.2d 788 (1976).
6. Marlene Industries Corp. v. Carnac Textiles, Inc., 45 N.Y.2d 327, 408 N.Y.S.2d 410 (1978).
7. Valmont Industries, Inc. v. Mitsui & Co. (U.S.A.), Inc., 419 F. Supp. 1238 (D. Neb. 1976).
8. N & D Fashions, Inc. v. DHJ Industries, Inc., 548 F.2d 722 (8th Cir. 1976).
9. S. Kornblum Metals Co. v. Intsel Corp., 38 N.Y.2d 376, 379 N.Y.S.2d 826 (1976).
10. Gaynor-Stafford Industries, Inc. v. Mafco Textures Fibers, 52 A.D.2d 481, 384 N.Y.S.2d 788 (1976).
11. U.C.C.§1-201(26).
12. Trailmobile Division of Pullman, Inc. v. Jones, 118 Ga. App. 472, 164 S.E.2d 346 (1968).
13. 297 F.2d 497 (1st Cir. 1962).
14. White, J. and Summers, R., *Uniform Commercial Code* p. 28-32 (2d ed. 1979).
15. C. Itoh & Co. v. Jordan International Co., 552 F.2d 1228 (7th Cir. 1977).
16. Steiner v. Mobil Oil Corp., 20 Cal. 3d 90, 141 Cal. Rptr. 157 (1977).
17. Southern Idaho Pipe & Steel Co. v. Cal-Cut Pipe & Supply, Inc., 98 Idaho 495, 567 P.2d 1246 (1977).
18. Uniroyal, Inc. v. Chambers Gasket & Mfg. Co., 380 N.E. 2d 571 (Ind. App. 1978).
19. Stoh v. Jordan, 552 F.2d 1228 (7th Cir. 1977).
20. Ibid. 1236.
21. White, J. and Summers, R., *Uniform Commercial Code* p. 38 (2d ed. 1979).
22. *Forms of Business Agreements and Resolutions.* 8116-5 (Institute for Business Planning, Inc. 1979).

General terms and conditions
listed on purchase order

Purchase Order
Name of Hospital-Vendee

To   Purchase Order No. _____

[   ]

(Vendor Name   Important
 and Address)   This purchase order number
                                                         must appear on all correspon-
[   ]   dence, invoices, packing slips,
                                                         shipping papers, and packag-
                                                         ing.

                                                         Date _____

Ship to: (Please Mail   Invoice To:
                      3 Copies of
[   ]   Invoice)   [   ]

(Receiving Dept.   (Accounts Payable
 of Vendee)   of Vendee)

[   ]   [   ]

Ship Via:	F.O.B.:	Payment Terms:	Delivery Required:
Dept.	Account No.	Notify:	Requisition No.

Furnish The Following Upon And Subject To All Conditions And Instructions Stated On Reverse Side.

Quantity	Description	Buyer Code	Price	Total

This order is not binding until accepted.

This order, including the terms and conditions on the face and reverse side hereof, contains the complete and final agreement between Buyer and Seller and no other agreement in any way modifying any of said terms and conditions will be binding upon Buyer unless made in writing and signed by Buyer's authorized representative.

Hospital/Vendee

By _____

Purchase Order is accepted <u>(Name of vendor)</u>, by _____.

On the reverse side of the purchase order, the Buyer should list the general terms and conditions under which every purchase is made. The following are representative of these terms or conditions the hospital-vendee may find advantageous to include in its purchase order.[22]

(1) *Acceptance*—This purchase order constitutes Buyer's offer to Seller, and commencement of performance pursuant to this Order shall constitute acceptance by Seller. Conditions stated by Seller in acknowledgment of this Order shall not affect Buyer's offer as represented by this Order, and shall not be binding on Buyer if in conflict with, or in addition to, any of the provisions of this Order (including delivery schedule, price, quantity, specifications, and terms and conditions) unless expressly agreed to in writing by Buyer.

(2) *Contract*—The contract resulting from the acceptance of this Order is to be construed according to the laws of the state from which this Order issues as shown by the address of the Buyer, which is printed on the face of this Order.

(3) *Delivery Schedules*—Deliveries are to be made at times specified by Buyer. If Seller fails to make deliveries at the time agreed upon, Buyer reserves the right to cancel, purchase elsewhere, and hold Seller accountable for any additional costs or damages incurred.

(4) *Excusable Delays*—Except with respect to defaults of subcontractors, Seller shall not be liable for delays or defaults in deliveries due to causes beyond its control and without its fault or negligence. If at any time Seller has reason to believe that deliveries will not be made as scheduled, written notice setting forth the cause of the anticipated delay will be given immediately to Buyer. Any delay due to default of subcontractor will be excusable if beyond the control and without the fault or negligence of both Seller and its subcontractor and if Seller establishes that it could not obtain supplies or services from any other source in time to meet the delivery schedule. Where the Buyer receives notification of a material or indefinite delay, he may by written notification to the Seller as to any delivery concerned, and where the prospective delay substantially impairs the value of the entire contract, then also as to the whole, either terminate and thereby discharge any unexecuted portion of the contract to modify the contract by agree-

ing to take available materials in substitution.

(5) *Prices*—Seller's price shall not be higher than last quoted or charged to Buyer unless otherwise agreed in writing. Invoices must be rendered for each shipment under this Order on date of shipment.

(6) *Taxes*—Except as may be otherwise provided in this Order, the price includes all applicable federal, state, and local taxes.

(7) *Quantities*—Shipments must equal exact amounts ordered. Unless agreed to by Buyer, Buyer will have no liability for payment for materials delivered to Buyer which are in excess of quantities specified on the face of the Order.

(8) *Warranty*—Seller expressly warrants that all the material and work covered by this Order will conform to the specifications, drawings, samples or other description furnished or specified by Buyer, and will be merchantable, of good material and workmanship and free from defect. Seller expressly warrants that all the material covered by this Order, which is the product of Seller or is in accordance with Seller's specifications, will be fit and sufficient for the purposes intended. This warranty shall survive any inspection, delivery, or acceptance of the materials, and payment therefor, by Buyer.

(9) *Inspection*—All material shall be received subject to Buyer's inspection and rejection. Defective material or material not in accordance with Buyer's specifications will be held for Seller's instruction and at Seller's risk and, if Seller so directs, will be returned at Seller's expense. No goods returned as defective shall be replaced without a new order and sched-ule. Payment for material on this Order prior to inspection shall not constitute an acceptance thereof, nor will acceptance remove Seller's responsibility for latent defects.

(10) *Patents*—By accepting this Order, Seller agrees to defend, protect, and save harmless Buyer, its successors, assigns, and users of its products, against all suits at law or in equity, and from all damages, claims, and demands, for actual or alleged infringement of any United States or foreign patent or copyright by reason of the use or sale of the material ordered.

(11) *Buyer's Property*—All material, including tools, furnished or specifically paid for by Buyer, shall be the property of Buyer, shall be subject to removal at any time without additional cost upon demand by Buyer, shall be used only in filling orders from Buyer, shall be kept separate from other materials or tools, and shall be clearly identified as the property of Buyer. Seller assumes all liability for loss or damage, with the exception of normal wear or tear, and agrees to supply detailed statements of inventory upon request of Buyer.

(12) *Tools*—Unless otherwise herein agreed, Seller at its own expense shall furnish, keep in good condition and replace when necessary all dies, tools, gauges, fixtures, patterns, etc., necessary for the production of the material ordered. The cost of changes in the aforementioned items necessary to effect design or specification changes ordered by Buyer shall be paid for by Buyer. Buyer has the option, however, to take possession of and title to any dies, tools, gauges, fixtures, patterns, etc., that are special for the production of the material covered by this Order and

shall pay to Seller the unamortized cost thereof; provided, however, that this option shall not apply if the material hereby ordered is the standard product of Seller or if a substantial quantity of like material is being sold by Seller to others.

(13) *Changes*—(a) Buyer may at any time, by a written order make changes within the general scope of this Order in any one or more of the following: (i) drawings, designs, or specifications (ii) method of shipment or packing; (iii) quantities of articles to be furnished; (iv) place of delivery; and (v) delivery schedules. If any such changes cause any increase or decrease in the cost of, or the item required for the performance of any part of the work under this Order, whether changed or not changed by any such order, an equitable adjustment shall be made in the price or delivery schedule, or both, and the Order shall be modified in writing accordingly. Any claim by Seller for adjustment under this clause must be asserted in writing within thirty (30) days from the date of receipt by Seller of the notification of change provided, however, that Buyer, if it decides that the facts justify such action, may receive and act upon any such claim asserted at any time prior to final payment under this Order. However, nothing in this clause shall excuse Seller from proceeding with this Order as changed. (b) Buyer's personnel may from time to time render assistance or give technical advice to, or exchange information with, Seller's personnel concerning this Order or the articles or services to be furnished hereunder. However, such assistance, advice statements, or exchange of information shall not constitute a waiver with respect to any of Seller's obligations or Buyer's rights hereunder, to be authority for any change in the articles called for hereunder. Any such waiver or change to be valid and binding upon Buyer must be in writing and signed by an authorized representative of Buyer's Purchasing Department. In case of any doubt, Seller should promptly consult Buyer's Purchasing Department for further instructions. (c) In connection with any claim for adjustment under this clause, Seller shall submit cost data in such form and detail as may reasonably be required by Buyer. (d) Where the cost of property made obsolete or excess as a result of a change is included in Seller's claim for adjustment pursuant to this clause, Buyer shall have the right to prescribe the manner of disposition of such property.

(14) *Supplementary Information*—Any specifications, drawings, notes, instructions, engineering notices, or technical data referred to in this Order shall be deemed to be incorporated herein by reference as if fully set forth. In case of any discrepancies or questions, refer to Buyer's Purchasing Department for decision or instructions or for interpretation.

(15) *Title to Drawings and Specifications*—Buyer shall at all times have title to all drawings and specifications furnished by Buyer to Seller and intended for use in connection with this Purchase Order. Seller shall use such drawings and specifications only in connection with this Order, and shall not disclose such drawings and specifications to any person, firm, or corporation other than Buyer's or Seller's employees, subcontractors, or Government inspectors. The Seller shall, upon

Buyer's request or upon completion of the Order, promptly return all drawings and specifications to Buyer.

(16) *Information Disclosed*—Unless otherwise expressly agreed to in writing by Buyer, no information or knowledge, heretofore or hereafter disclosed to Buyer, in the performance of or in connection with this Order, shall be deemed to be confidential or proprietary, and any such information or knowledge shall be free from any restrictions (other than claim for patent infringement) as part of the consideration for this Order.

(17) *Shipping and Billing*—(a) All material shall be suitably packed, marked, and shipped in accordance with the requirements of common carriers in a manner to secure lowest transportation cost and no additional charge shall be made to the Buyer therefor unless otherwise stated herein. (b) No charge shall be made by Seller for drayage or storage, unless otherwise stated herein. (c) Seller shall properly mark each package with Buyer's order number and where multiple packages comprise a single shipment each package shall also be consecutively numbered. Purchase order number and package numbers shall be shown on packing slips, bills of lading, and invoices. (d) Packing slips must accompany each shipment. (e) Original bill of lading, or other shipment receipt, for each shipment shall be attached to the invoice and promptly forwarded by Seller. (f) Seller agrees to describe material on bill of lading or other shipping receipt and to route shipment in accordance with instructions issued by Buyer. (g) Render invoices in duplicate on day of shipment accompanied by bill of lading. (h) Monthly statements must be rendered promptly.

(18) *Title and Delivery of Goods*—When goods are purchased FOB Seller's plant or shipping point, it is agreed between Seller and Buyer that the goods covered by this Order shall not be considered as delivered and title thereto shall not pass until the goods reach the Buyer's receiving point indicated hereon. However, Buyer assumes responsibility at the FOB point for carrier routing, transportation charges, and risk of loss or damages to the goods in transit.

(19) *State Approval of Vehicle Equipment*—If the articles covered by this purchase order require approval for the sale and/or use thereof by a state statute or regulation, Seller certifies it has or will obtain an approval for their sale and/or use from the appropriate agency of each of the states requiring same, and upon request, Seller will submit to Buyer a photostat of each such approval for sale and/or use.

(20) *Duty Drawback Rights*—This purchase order includes all related customs, duty, and import drawback rights, if any (including rights developed by substitution and rights which may be acquired from Seller's suppliers), which Seller can transfer to Buyer. Seller agrees to inform Buyer of the existence of any such rights and upon request to supply such documents as may be required to obtain such drawback.

(21) *Government Regulations*—In the performance of work under this Order, Seller agrees to comply with all applicable federal, state, or local laws, rules, regulations, or ordinances.

(22) *Insolvency*—Buyer may forthwith

cancel the contract resulting from the acceptance of this Order in the event of the happening of any of the following, or of any other comparable event: Insolvency of the Seller: The filing of a voluntary petition of bankruptcy: The filing of an involuntary petition to have Seller declared bankrupt provided it is not vacated within thirty (30) days from the date of filing: The appointment of a receiver or trustee for Seller provided such appointment is not vacated within thirty (30) days from the date of such appointment: The execution by Seller of an assignment for the benefit of creditors.

(23) *Advertising*—Seller shall not, without first obtaining the written consent of Buyer, in any manner, advertise or publish the fact that Seller has contracted to furnish Buyer the material herein ordered, and for failure to observe this provision, Buyer shall have the right to terminate the contract resulting from the acceptance of this order without any obligation to accept deliveries after the date of termination or make further payments except for completed articles delivered prior to termination.

(24) *Assignment*—Neither this Order nor any interest under it shall be assigned by Seller without the prior written consent of Buyer, except the claims for monies due or to become due under this Order may be assigned by Seller without such consent, and subject to the provisions of this paragraph. Buyer shall promptly be furnished with two signed copies of any such assignment. Payment to an assignee of any such claim shall be subject to setoff or recoupment for any present or future claim or claims which Buyer may have against Seller, except to the extent that any such claims may be expressly waived in writing by Buyer. Buyer reserves the right to make direct settlements and/or adjustments in price(s) with Seller, notwithstanding any assignment of claims for monies due or to become due hereunder and without notice to the assignee.

(25) *Remedies*—The remedies herein reserved shall be cumulative, and additional to any other or further remedies provided in law or equity. No waiver of a breach of any provision of this contract shall constitute a waiver of any other breach, or of such provision.

Simplifying the purchase procedure

Richard L. Pinkerton, Ph.D.
Dean
Graduate School of Administration
Capital University
Columbus, Ohio

FAR TOO MANY hospital buyers spend too much time and paperwork on repetitive small orders. Consequently, they have greatly reduced opportunities to work on complex, critical procurement problems, such as inventory control, purchase of expensive capital equipment, long-term contracts, and value analysis. Many purchasing or materiel managers identify solving the small order problem as a major problem for most purchasing departments. Much, however, can be accomplished by simplifying that part of the purchasing process that does indeed involve the "simple." There are major basic techniques and methods available to help solve or reduce the cost and frustration involved with small orders, orders that take time but save few resources for the hospital. After what can be simplified is determined, paperwork techniques, internal procedures, and external contracting methods can be applied in solving the small order problem. (See Table 1.)

Table 1. Simplifying the purchase process

Identifying the Small Order Value Problem
Complexity of the purchase: straight rebuy, mod-
ified rebuy, new buy
How much is it worth? ABC inventory analysis

Simplifying Paperwork Techniques
Traveling requisitions
Combination requisition-purchase order
Self-invoice forms
Purchase order draft
Short form limited purchase order
Magnetic cards
Flex-O-Writer
Word processing

Simplifying Internal Purchasing Procedures
Petty cash
Telephone orders
Designated purchasing days and laundry lists
Centralized purchasing
Post-purchase buyer appraisal of invoices

External Contracting Methods
Blanket orders
Systems contracts
Stockless purchasing
Group purchasing
Consignment buying

IDENTIFYING THE PROBLEM

Before purchasing procedures can be simplified or their costs reduced, the question of "what to simplify" must be addressed. One good technique for categorizing the purchases of any operation is to classify the purchased items according to the complexity of the purchase.[1]

Straight Rebuy

This category includes rather standardized and often undifferentiated goods that are automatically reordered at a reorder point, determined by a physical count or a time period. An example is surgical tape with no changed specifications, available from several previously used vendors. When the X package is opened, the tape is reordered using a traveling requisition (TR) that has predetermined specifications, quantities, and alternative vendors from a qualified vendor list. The TR is simply a reusable or repeating requisition that goes back and forth between the user and the buyer. Although the TR itself is a time-saver, the real value of the straight rebuy classification is in identifying a group of goods that can be reviewed for rather automatic buying procedures.

Modified Rebuy

This category covers items purchased before but for which the specifications or "needs" may have changed enough to call in a vendor for help. Changes could include such buying considerations as contract terms, delivery dates, price, standards, and others beyond changes in physical-functional characteristics. This category of goods is also a candidate for simplification but less so than straight rebuy goods.

New Buy

These items are either goods that have never been purchased before or items that call for extensive problem solving, such as major equipment, services, and new contract terms. By reducing the time spent on the first two categories, buyers can devote more effort where it is needed in such areas as complicated procurement, commodity analysis, price-cost analysis, sources, vendor evaluation, inventory control, value analysis, and other high payoff aspects of materiel management.

ABC ANALYSIS

Another classical breakdown of commodities other than traditional ones such as maintenance, repairs, and operating (MRO), raw materials, and capital equipment is the ABC inventory-commodity analysis.[2] This concept classifies past purchases according to number of items vs. dollar value and is based on last year's commodity record. Table 2 shows the ABC classification of items by percentage of total physical volume and dollar volume.

This analysis identifies the high-value items, the A category, and the very low-value items, the C category; it is the C category and perhaps the B category that offers the greatest opportunities for automation and simplification, thus freeing valuable time to concentrate on the products that must be constantly managed relative to need, price, and inventory position.

The easiest method to arrive at the ABC breakdown involves listing categories or ranges of dollar values by range of number of items followed by a simple percentage breakdown. This is a simple task using a computer or even manual manipulation.

It is now rather apparent that the automatic or semiautomatic purchases or the straight rebuys and modified rebuys and the B and C items are the types to investigate for possible simplification of purchasing procedures. There are three major areas to examine: (1) paperwork techniques and flow; (2) internal procedures; and (3) external contracting methods.

SIMPLIFYING TECHNIQUES AND METHODS

Paperwork Techniques

Reduced documentation for repetitive purchasing should be one of the objectives. The following techniques have proved successful in this regard.

TRAVELING REQUISITIONS

The TR, a reusable requisition device, is a purchase history card containing predetermined vendors, quantities, specifications, pricing, and inventory data. When the item is to be ordered, the inventory record card is pulled and the TR is sent to purchasing for ordering. It is then returned to the user, saving requisition preparation as well as order time.

COMBINATION REQUISITION-PURCHASE ORDER FORM

With this form, the requisitioner in effect writes the purchase order since one section contains the requesting data and the other part contains the order data. (See Figure 1.) Caution must be used to avoid complicating this form. The purchase of simple items must not be "overcontrolled" and other data must be kept to the minimum, such as description, account-budget line identification, price, quantity, delivery date, vendor block, signature blocks for

Table 2. The ABC classification system

	Physical Count	Dollar Volume
A items	20 (5%)	70 (80%)
B items	10 (15%)	10 (15%)
C items	70 (80%)	20 (5%)
Total	100 (100%)	100 (100%)

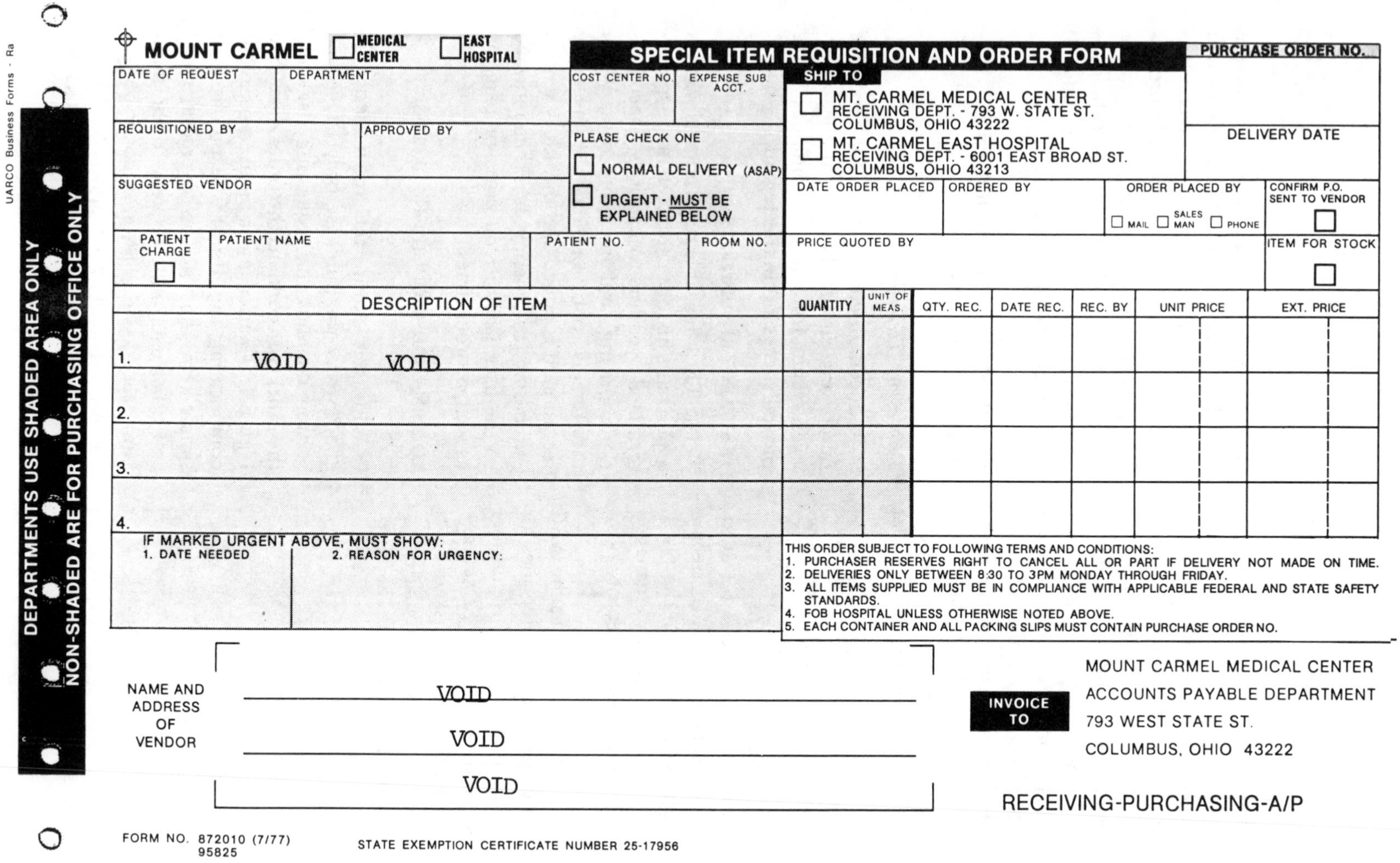

UARCO Business Forms - Ra

DEPARTMENTS USE SHADED AREA ONLY
NON-SHADED ARE FOR PURCHASING OFFICE ONLY

MOUNT CARMEL ☐ MEDICAL CENTER ☐ EAST HOSPITAL

SPECIAL ITEM REQUISITION AND ORDER FORM

PURCHASE ORDER NO.

DATE OF REQUEST | DEPARTMENT | COST CENTER NO. | EXPENSE SUB ACCT.

SHIP TO
☐ MT. CARMEL MEDICAL CENTER
RECEIVING DEPT. - 793 W. STATE ST.
COLUMBUS, OHIO 43222
☐ MT. CARMEL EAST HOSPITAL
RECEIVING DEPT. - 6001 EAST BROAD ST.
COLUMBUS, OHIO 43213

DELIVERY DATE

REQUISITIONED BY | APPROVED BY

PLEASE CHECK ONE
☐ NORMAL DELIVERY (ASAP)
☐ URGENT - MUST BE EXPLAINED BELOW

SUGGESTED VENDOR

DATE ORDER PLACED | ORDERED BY | ORDER PLACED BY ☐ MAIL ☐ SALES MAN ☐ PHONE | CONFIRM P.O. SENT TO VENDOR ☐

PATIENT CHARGE ☐ | PATIENT NAME | PATIENT NO. | ROOM NO.

PRICE QUOTED BY | ITEM FOR STOCK ☐

DESCRIPTION OF ITEM	QUANTITY	UNIT OF MEAS.	QTY. REC.	DATE REC.	REC. BY	UNIT PRICE	EXT. PRICE
1. VOID VOID							
2.							
3.							
4.							

IF MARKED URGENT ABOVE, MUST SHOW:
1. DATE NEEDED
2. REASON FOR URGENCY:

THIS ORDER SUBJECT TO FOLLOWING TERMS AND CONDITIONS:
1. PURCHASER RESERVES RIGHT TO CANCEL ALL OR PART IF DELIVERY NOT MADE ON TIME.
2. DELIVERIES ONLY BETWEEN 8:30 TO 3PM MONDAY THROUGH FRIDAY.
3. ALL ITEMS SUPPLIED MUST BE IN COMPLIANCE WITH APPLICABLE FEDERAL AND STATE SAFETY STANDARDS.
4. FOB HOSPITAL UNLESS OTHERWISE NOTED ABOVE.
5. EACH CONTAINER AND ALL PACKING SLIPS MUST CONTAIN PURCHASE ORDER NO.

NAME AND ADDRESS OF VENDOR
VOID
VOID
VOID

INVOICE TO
MOUNT CARMEL MEDICAL CENTER
ACCOUNTS PAYABLE DEPARTMENT
793 WEST STATE ST.
COLUMBUS, OHIO 43222

RECEIVING-PURCHASING-A/P

FORM NO. 872010 (7/77)
95825

STATE EXEMPTION CERTIFICATE NUMBER 25-17956

Figure 1. Special item requisition and order form. (Reprinted with permission.)

requisitioner, and buyer and purchase order number. The buyer's signature converts the requisition into an order.[3]

There are many business form suppliers with standard (and less costly) forms to select from as opposed to designing one. Ordinary commercial printers should be avoided because they will simply subcontract the work to a forms printer for an additional 10 to 20 percent "add on" to the price; it is preferable to order directly from a forms printer.

SELF-INVOICE FORMS

Some suppliers provide snap-out forms that contain copies for billing, inspection-receiving, purchasing, the requisitioner, etc. If the suppliers for miscellaneous and other minor items are not providing this service, it might be a good subject for the next negotiating session.

PURCHASE ORDER DRAFT

Kaiser Aluminum Company pioneered the technique of attaching a previously prepared blank check with limits for full shipments and dollar restrictions. Although it saves time for accounts payable there is no savings for the purchasing department, but purchase order drafts do help reduce the total procurement cost, which includes payment preparation. Although the check-purchase combination is rarely used, the buyer may be able to negotiate lower prices, better service, and faster delivery simply because the vendor receives immediate payment.

SHORT FORM OR LIMITED PURCHASE ORDER FORM

This is a simplified purchase order form usually limited to a small-dollar amount with no backorders allowed and using a separate set of purchase order control numbers. It is usually prepared by the user department and sent directly to the vendor with a copy to purchasing.

MAGNETIC CARDS

A wide variety of automated memory typewriters that use magnetic cards to store a format, such as a purchase order form, are available. An example is the IBM Office System 6, Mag Card II Typewriter. With or without visual display, this equipment allows simultaneous typing and form preparation, usually with a storage capacity for recall of purchasing data. IBM and other manufacturers offer many options, including direct access to computers, but full office systems belong to the word processing category.

FLEX-O-WRITER

Although it is now obsolete, some firms still use a special electric typewriter that will produce a purchase order from prepared tapes or edge-punched cards. These tapes can also be used to "feed" a computer for a variety of purchasing reports.[4]

WORD PROCESSING

Automated office systems will eventually be applied to purchasing but the present systems are so new that there is very little experience with them in the field of materiel management. Several firms now offer memory typewriting equipment with instant correction via an electronic display with the completed work fed into a memory storage unit with optional printout capacity.

Word processing offers enormous clerical time-saving possibilities in purchasing and is a natural addition to existing computerized purchase order preparation systems. When word processing is combined with cathode ray tube (CRT) instant retrieval display screens, purchasing paperwork will be greatly reduced.[5]

A simple IBM Mag Card II Typewriter unit costs approximately $8,900 or $283 per month on lease; more sophisticated systems such as the IBM Office System 6-6/452 Information Processor cost approximately $19,000 or $600 per month on lease. When the application is correct, the savings in reduced paperwork and flow time can more than offset the costs of the automated office. It should be noted that these systems can have various purchasing forms in their memory units. The high-density storage diskettes available with IBM's Office System 6 allow substantial memory storage, an excellent method for monitoring various purchasing-inventory reports. These systems are also compatible with magnetic cards so that mag cards can be prepared by users on mag typewriters and sent to purchasing or central inventory control.

SIMPLIFYING INTERNAL PURCHASING PROCEDURES

Petty Cash

User departments often keep a few hundred dollars in petty cash for direct purchases requiring only the receipts signed by a buyer. This allows "lunch time" procurement by the user at approved vendors. A safer variation of this system is authorized credit cards established for certain vendors, with limits on dollar

Word processing offers enormous clerical time-saving possibilities and is a natural addition to existing computerized purchase order preparation systems.

amounts. Many maintenance departments use this procedure and even a few office managers have accounts at discount stores for single-quantity items of limited value.

Of course, the petty cash account can be controlled by the purchasing department, but the key to workability is prior approval of certain local vendors and establishment of dollar and quantity limits. The point is that $25 in elaborate paperwork should not be spent to buy a $10 item.

Telepone Orders

Every purchasing department uses or should use telephone orders. Although many such orders must be followed up with a confirming purchase order, especially those requiring a written document such as a contract for $500 or more of goods, services, and one year or more of performance, not every order should be reduced to a contract. For the low-value, simple small orders from local suppliers, a telephone log book can be kept with the date, items, price, quantity, and delivery date.

Designated Purchasing Days and Laundry Lists

Orders for specific commodities can be scheduled for particular days. For example, all miscellaneous small-order supplies of one type can be ordered on Wednesday, no later than 12:00 PM for a prearranged Wednesday afternoon pick-up by the vendor. The requisition can simply be attached to one order file or can be made on preprinted forms with or without specifications, often called a "laundry list."[6] The "laundry list" may also consist of nothing more than line-by-line items that are duplicated by the buyer and given to the vendor's pick-up and delivery person, who deposits last week's order and picks up the new order.

These techniques eliminate the daily preparation of small orders by establishing special depository trays in the buying office, which enables a secretary to "file" the request for pick-up on the designated day.

Centralized Purchasing

All repetitious orders should be consolidated to avoid unnecessary orders over short time periods. Care must be taken to avoid having two different departments ordering different brands or only slightly different specifications of the same material. Past commodity analysis can help identify candidates for consolidation and other standardization projects.[7]

Post-Purchase Buyer Approval of Invoices

This procedure is a slight variation of petty cash purchasing and can be called "direct requisitioner purchasing." Some institutions are allowing more "unique" and single, small-quantity items to be purchased directly as long as no consolidation is possible. In this procedure, the buyer merely signs the invoice.

Direct purchase has much merit for institutions operating on a department-by-department preapproved line-item budget. If department heads have already had their budgets approved, they are then authorized to make the expenditure. The remaining task in purchasing is to get the most for the money. Once purchasing has selected the vendor for small-volume or minimum-order items of a general nature, such as floor sealer, direct telephone purchase with limits established with the vendor according to a monthly percentage of budget can be authorized. The vendor should ship only orders phoned or picked up by preselected authorized individuals in the particular department.

EXTERNAL CONTRACTING METHODS

Blanket Orders

This is probably the oldest simplifying technique and involves negotiating a long-term contract for a particular item that has a rather large annual usage but that must be shipped in smaller amounts on a regular basis. To avoid repetitious orders of the same material from either a single or multiple vendor list, the buyer consolidates the forecasted usage, usually over a 6- to 12-month period, with planned releases for a particular delivery schedule per week, per month, or as otherwise required.[8]

The purchase order contract should specify price; specifications; delivery dates, including a forecasted release schedule; quality standards; cancellation procedures; and any other special clauses, such as price-change warning and warranty-breach provisions. The goal is to establish a firm fixed price, but in today's inflationary economy, the vendor may insist on a price redetermination clause, such as escalator provisions tied to a predetermined index, e.g., the wholesale price index (WPI) found in various government publications, or other such indices from various government publications.

The long-term purchase contract offers an opportunity for the buyer to negotiate a price-change warning clause specifying, for example, 60 days' notice, no later than the fifteenth of each month, in writing and with documentation to justify the price increase requested by the vendor. Depending on the total volume, the buyer may want to split the business into equal portions with three vendors or with one vendor for maximum volume discount.

A variation of the blanket order device is the requirements contract in which buyers simply order at one time all of their purchase needs for a definite future period, with the purchase order covering the same details as listed earlier. Great care must be exercised in the contract wording to avoid legal difficulties, and words such as "may use" might not be sufficient to determine "consideration," one of the key requirements necessary for a valid contract.[9]

Whatever the form used, the release may be executed by phone, written form, or computer and then recorded with the original blanket order contract.

Systems Contracts

A variation of the blanket order, the systems contract, is more sophisticated and involves subcontracting an entire class of goods to one vendor.[10] The most common example of this type of contracting is offered by American Hospital Supply, a division of American Hospital

Whatever the form used, the release may be executed by phone, written form or computer and then recorded with the original blanket order contract.

Supply Corporation, which sells a system called Analytical Systems Automated Purchasing (ASAP). Use of ASAP has now expanded to the entire range of the MRO class of goods.

In ASAP, all systems contracts should go through the following preparation cycle.

The buyer tabulates last year's purchases and forecasts the next year's requirements. This analysis must be done line-item by line-item with a quantity and price for each commodity and the location of use.

Armed with this purchase history and future needs, the buyer now calls in three or four of the best local distributors and manufacturers, and in separate negotiations gives these data to the potential vendors.

The buyer then asks the prospective suppliers to prepare proposals for the entire family of goods. These proposals should include a master catalogue of the items with prices for certain volumes, the inventory availability of each item, delivery time, and other contract clauses such as those described under blanket orders.

Most suppliers will offer an automatic ordering system, using some form of data phone. A data phone is a direct order device that uses telephone lines and is usually tied to a perpetual inventory record system. A buyer then can order direct from the supplier via teletype by using a toll-free number that gives access to the supplier's order preparation equipment. Some suppliers also offer a print-back terminal that produces multiple copies of the packing slip for each order, usually in 8 to 10 minutes. The rental charges to the buyer vary from $40 to $125 per month for the Bell Telephone transmitting equipment. Monthly or other periodic order-inventory status reports are available.

Controls can be built into the system to limit the order quantities, and invoicing is usually on a monthly basis. Although most hospitals have one transmitter, for larger complexes several can be installed to allow direct purchase by the requisitioner. Multiple copies of the master catalog can be placed with major using departments.

During negotiation sessions after the proposals are received, the buyer bargains for maximum price and service advantages. In return for all of the business and assuming legality under the Robinson-Patman Act, the buyer should receive substantial discounts versus past prices obtained under a small order condition.[11]

Other safety features can be incorporated into the systems contract, such as maximum delivery times and requirements for the vendor to supply the items if stock outs occur by obtaining the goods from a backup vendor.

The buyer awards the contract to one supplier with provisions for cancellation.

The buyer must monitor the records since this is critical in watching for price changes and ordering quantities over budgeted amounts, i.e., variance analysis. The contract must be reviewed at least yearly or at the agreed reopener time in the contract. Although systems contracts have the obvious disadvantage of single source, the reduction in paperwork cost is enormous; in addition, they allow the release of valuable buyer time and reduced prices through large-volume buys. It should be noted that data phone systems can be used without systems contracts, but only where the volume justifies the rental cost.

Stockless Purchasing

In return for sizable orders, many vendors will agree to "hold" a certain level of inventory, thereby saving the inventory cost which is at least 30 percent of the average inventory value. As Charles E. Housley writes, laboratory and radiology are excellent departments to implement the concept since these departments have well-defined specifications and the least amount of items.[12] Central stores inventories only standardized items used by several departments or requisition areas.

Group Purchasing

If a collection of hospitals can agree on standardized items, consolidated ordering can produce significant savings. The Chicago Hospital Council; the Hospital Bureau in Pleasantville, New York; and Sisters of Mercy Hospitals operated by the Sisters' Chicago and Detroit Provinces are excellent examples.[13]

These groups usually form a central buying office to handle negotiations of blanket orders, systems contracts, etc., and the trade-off of this expense is measured by the savings involved in lower prices and lower purchasing preparation time in each hospital.

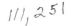

Vendors have not been receptive to the idea of group purchasing because of the obvious increased power to the buyer. Some purchasing agents and users resent the loss of control and necessity for standardization. These are hardly legitimate reasons to oppose group buying efforts. Although such efforts must be careful not to violate federal and state anticollusion and discrimination laws that attempt to avoid restraint of trade, group purchasing has enough successful examples to warrant serious consideration, especially in this time of close examination of hospital costs.[14]

Consignment Buying

What is not used can be returned. Some vendors ship but only invoice as the material is used; i.e., as each carton is opened, the buyer owns the goods. The savings include less inventory cost and reduced order activity because larger safety stocks can be ordered if there is storage room.

Once the buyer has identified the highly repetitive items of rather low value by using the complexity analysis and ABC inventory breakdown, specific paperwork flow, internal procedures, and external contracting methods can be applied to the most appropriate items or classes of purchased goods.

Internal procedures and external contracting methods can be applied to the most appropriate items or classes of purchased goods.

The advantages of using these simplifying methods are:
- greatly reduced paperwork;
- fast flow from requisition to delivery;
- reduced unit prices;
- better delivery and increased satisfaction from users;
- better terms; and
- released buyer time for more sophisticated procurement and materiel management projects such as community services, price-cost analysis, price trends, inventory control procedures, vendor visitation, selection, vendor evaluation, forecasting of materiel needs, contract negotiations, value analysis, and so on.

More advantages could be cited; all help reduce the administrative cost of purchasing and the absolute cost of the items purchased. Not all the methods will work in any particular hospital, but they should be investigated for better purchasing with fewer dollars.

REFERENCES

1. Robinson, P. J., Faris, C. W., and Wind, Y. *Industrial Buying and Creative Marketing* (Boston: The Marketing Science Institute and Allyn F. Bacon, Inc. 1967) p. 28.
2. England, W. B. and Leenders, M. R. *Purchasing and Materials Management* 6th ed. (Homewood, Ill.: Richard D. Irwin, Inc. 1975) p. 356-357.
3. Rourke, R. E. "Handling Small Orders Fast With a Requisition/Purchase Order Form." *Purchasing Administration* 4:1 (January-February 1980) p. 2-3, 34. See also: Baker, J., Kuehne, R. S., McCoy, D. and Witter, Jr., D. M. *Purchasing Factomatic: A Portfolio of Successful Forms, Reports, Records, and Procedures* (Englewood Cliffs, N.J.: Prentice-Hall 1977).
4. Westing, J. H., Fine, J. V., and Zenz, G. J. *Purchasing Management: Materials in Motion* 4th ed. (New

York: John Wiley & Sons, Inc. 1976) p. 477.

5. "Information Processing and Tomorrow's Office." *Fortune* (October 8, 1979) p. 31-70. (A special advertisement-article section prepared by the International Data Corporation).

6. Dowst, S. "Short-Cut Systems Pull Together for Long Haul." *Purchasing Magazine* (September 26, 1979) p. 95. Also see by the same author *More Basics for Buyers* Available from CBI Publishing Co., 51 Sleeper St., Boston, Mass. 02210.

7. Corey, R. E. "Should Companies Centralize Procurement?" *Harvard Business Review* 56:6 (Nov.-Dec. 1978) p. 102-110.

8. Lee, Jr., L. and Dobler, D. W. *Purchasing and Materials Management: Text and Cases* 3rd ed. (New York: McGraw-Hill Book Co. 1977) p. 428-429.

9. Wiesner, D. A. "Requirements Contract: By Accident or Design?" *Journal of Purchasing and Materials Management* 13:4 (Winter 1977) p. 6-9. Available from The National Association of Purchasing Management, 11 Park Place, New York, N.Y., 10007.

10. Ammer, D. S. *Profit-Conscious Purchasing: A Treasury of Newly Developed Cost-Reduction Buying Methods* (Chicago: The Dartnell Corp. 1977) p. 268-274.

11. Murray, J. E., Jr. *Purchasing and the Law* (Pittsburgh: Purchasing Management Association, Inc. 1973) p. 100-108. Available from Purchasing Management Association, P.O. Box 9306, Pittsburgh, Pa., 15225. Also see Murray, J. E., Jr. "Supreme Backing for Tough Negotiating." *Purchasing World* (May 1979) p. 37.

12. Housley, C. E. *Hospital Materiel Management* (Germantown, Md.: Aspen Systems Corp. 1978) p. 197-201 as reprinted from "Stockless Purchasing Makes Dollars and Sense." *Dimensions in Health Service* 54:5 (May 1977) p. 24-26.

13. Ammer, D. S. *Purchasing and Materials Management for Health Care Institutions* (Toronto: Lexington Books, D.C. Heath and Company 1975) p. 79-83.

14. Ammer, *Purchasing and Materials Management for Health Care Institutions*, p. 79-83.

Total centralized purchasing: can it ever be achieved?

S. Randolph Hayas
Consultant
Health Care Services Group
Ernst and Whinney
Cleveland, Ohio

THE HOSPITAL administrator may be overlooking one of the most effective ways to control nonwage expenses and improve internal control of the purchasing function by not evaluating, supporting and enforcing centralized purchasing.

In the past ten years hospitals have experienced annual expenditure increases ranging from 11 to 18 percent. In all cases this annual "inflation" rate has surpassed the overall general rate of inflation in the United States economy—in certain years nearly doubling. This has caused increased interest by the federal government to control increases in the health care segment of the economy. In this effort cost-containment bills have been proposed which are intended to check cost increases.

In 1977 the health care industry responded to government pressure and established the Voluntary Effort (VE). The American Hospital Association, the American Medical Association and the Federation of American Hospitals formed a National Steering Committee in 1977 to oversee and implement the VE. Although these three organizations are the major forces behind VE, there are many other participants. The main program objective is to reduce the annual increase in national hospital expenditures by two percent in 1978 and 1979. Cost-containment bills are waiting in the wings to apply mandatory controls if the VE does not achieve results.

In addition to government intervention, the hospital administrator and governing board must weigh the impact of large rate increases on the community the hospital serves. Thus the hospital is being pressured from both the federal government and the local community causing the hospital to earnestly search for ways to control costs. One option which many hospitals are undertaking is centralized purchasing.

WHAT IS CENTRALIZED PURCHASING?

Centralized purchasing is defined as centralizing the responsibility and authority for the hospital-wide purchasing function under one manager. In many hospitals this is drastically different from the current situation.

In definition, centralized purchasing is quite specific, but in fact there are varying degrees of "centralization" within hospitals. While some hospitals do practice nearly true centralized purchasing, others permit the purchasing of specialized items used by one department (e.g., pharmaceuticals, food) by that department head.

ADVANTAGES OF CENTRALIZED PURCHASING

Centralized purchasing, when properly established and enforced, allows for both cost savings and improved internal control of the procurement function. Its most common advantages (benefits) include the following.

- Quantity discounts are made possible by consolidating all hospital orders for the same and similar items.
- Product evaluation and standardization efforts are possible.
- Fewer purchase orders are processed thereby reducing purchasing, receiving and inspection time. This also reduces recordkeeping and makes that recordkeeping more effective.
- Duplication of effort and poor purchasing practices are minimized through coordination of purchases.
- Purchasing specialists whose primary responsibility is purchasing are developed.
- Department heads are able to devote full efforts to their main responsibilities (i.e., managing their department rather than ordering their department's supplies).
- The number of employees involved in purchasing is reduced.
- The purchasing manager is held accountable by the hospital administrator for the purchasing function.
- The hospital can maximize participation in a group purchasing program due to an increased knowledge of the hospital's needs.
- A unified purchasing policy can be developed.

- Centralized purchasing can attract a high quality purchasing professional because of the opportunities and challenges.

In a typical centralized purchasing environment the purchasing department usually buys for:

- general service departments (those departments that provide service to other departments and do not generate patient revenue);
- nursing care areas (including medical/surgical and special care units); and
- ancillary departments.

OBSTACLES TO CENTRALIZING PURCHASING

The departments that are most difficult to commit to centralized purchasing are those that feel they require too high a level of technical competence for a buyer to procure their equipment and supplies. These departments feel that because of this necessary high level of technical knowledge only they can adequately procure their needs. Departments that are typically most difficult to commit to the concept of centralized purchasing are:

- pharmacy;
- food service;

Departments that are most difficult to commit to centralized purchasing are those that feel they require too high a level of technical competence for a buyer to procure their equipment and supplies.

- maintenance; and
- certain ancillary departments such as radiology or laboratory.

Although department heads may feel their purchases are too technical for a purchasing specialist to perform, through adequately written specifications the purchasing agent can procure at least as effectively as the department head. The unwillingness to spend time putting into writing the required specifications for an item may be one of the major reasons for a department's reluctance to agree to centralized purchasing.

HOW TO ESTABLISH CENTRALIZED PURCHASING

The three essential steps to effectively accomplish centralized purchasing are (1) obtaining full hospital administrative support, (2) "selling" the benefits to department heads to receive their cooperation and (3) establishing the purchasing department's credibility through a slow yet steady implementation process.

Obtaining Administrative Support

As in any other hospital policy modification, the first step is to obtain the hospital administration's full agreement and support. Administrative support cannot be overemphasized in its importance since a change to centralized purchasing can be very traumatic to certain department heads causing them to search for ways to circumvent the new purchasing system. In addition, methods to control and enforce the policy should be established. These could include issuing no purchase orders except from the purchasing department and allowing no invoices to be paid by the accounts payable department without a properly authorized purchase order.

Selling the Benefits

Selling centralized purchasing to all departments may be the greatest task since many department heads enjoy the interaction with vendors or the ability that currently exists to order supplies at any time without any prepurchase planning efforts (e.g., establishing reorder points, defining in writing the product specifications, etc.).

Department heads must obtain a complete understanding of centralized purchasing in order for them not to feel threatened by this impending change. It must be understood that centralized purchasing is a method to relieve department heads from purchasing functions in order to spend more time where their specialized talents can be best utilized—managing their department. Furthermore, through proper planning and the establishment of well-defined, written product specifications, reorder points, order quantities and inventory levels, the supply flow should be no less consistent than prior to centralized purchasing and in most cases improvements should occur.

Establishing Credibility

After the hospital administration and department heads are sold on the concept and agree to work toward its accomplishment, reasonable goals and objectives should be established. The goals estab-

lished should specifically state dates for implementing the centralized purchasing plan in each department, the date for full centralized purchasing implementation within the hospital, and the savings and other improvements anticipated. It is important to prepare a timetable for implementation of the purchasing program to minimize procrastination on the part of purchasing, hospital administration and other departments.

One department should be chosen as the first area to implement centralized purchasing. It would not be practical to begin on "January 1" a complete (hospital-wide) centralized purchasing program; rather one department should be worked with to define items, specifications, substitutes, vendors, inventory levels, lead times, reorder points, order quantities and appropriate ordering patterns. Often a traveling requisition type card (containing the necessary purchasing information) is most effective for transmitting a purchase request from the requesting department to the purchasing department.

Often the best department to begin the implementation is laboratory or radiology. Many of the supplies in these departments may currently be procured through purchasing and often a good relationship exists between purchasing and the department to easily facilitate the change. The pharmacy department in most cases will be the most difficult in which to implement centralized purchasing. When centralized purchasing has been implemented in one department and is fully functional, another department should be chosen for the implementation process.

As centralized purchasing is implemented in each department, ongoing reviews should be conducted of the function of centralized purchasing to identify weaknesses and improvements. This review should be augmented by performance reporting by the purchasing department and by internal and oftentimes objective external audits of the purchasing function. The reviews, performance reporting and audits should be continued peri-odically after all departments have been fully implemented.

Centralized purchasing can be achieved, but it will take a sincere effort by hospital administration, all department heads and the purchasing department with the purchasing manager being the one to initiate the feasibility of centralized purchasing.

Mere purchasing versus effective negotiation

Martin G. Wooldridge
Director
Material Management
Regina General Hospital
Regina, Saskatchewan
Canada

THE CONTRASTS between mere purchasing and effective negotiation are easily discernible and can have immense impact on the benefits that an institution can accrue and the value of the contribution that materiel-purchasing personnel can make. Negotiation techniques, however, have not traditionally been major tools in the health care materiel environment. Contributory factors have included historic reliance on purchasing conventions that have stated that products when tendered should be accepted on the basis of the "first price being the best price" and the assumption that it is in some way unethical to request further benefits from the preferred supplier.

Institutions that are owned or controlled by city, county, state, or federal government agencies have often been subjected to tendering regulations that call for public disclosure of bids. This practice creates great pressure for the tendering organization to accept the lowest total price, without any additional benefits being secured other than those to be complied with as requested in the original tender documents.

NEGOTIATION PREREQUISITES

The benefits that are now well documented from the creation of major contract item consolidations with prime vendor arrangements[1] could not be achieved by the traditional purchasing technique of selecting the lowest individual item price from a multi-item tender list or even by choosing the vendor with the lowest total list calculation.

Initially the materiel-purchasing professional should determine the minimum objectives to be attained from a particular tendering exercise, and these should be the subject of a series of clear unequivocal statements in the tender request document. (See Appendices A and B.) It will then be clearly understood by all participating vendors that the personnel representing the institution can be expected to hold further discussions with at least some of the participants to clarify or increase the scope of some aspects of the vendor offer.

Institutional policies and procedures relating to purchasing practices must be revised, when necessary, to categorically indicate that all contract submissions will be regarded as strictly confidential and that the buyer reserves the right to reject the lowest or any bid. (See Appendices B and C.) This is an essential element in providing a suitable framework for the practice of negotiation techniques. Purchasing personnel who are unfamiliar with negotiation skills may generate confusion in the participating vendor community by disclosing participating vendor pricing and terms to direct competitors and thus creating a flurry of supplementary proposals from all sources.

The result is that the purchaser is now presiding over a "bidding war" and has essentially lost control of a project that requires firm guidance and direction to attain the predetermined objectives. The vendor position is that the buyer's objectives are no longer discernible and that all familiar tendering conventions have collapsed. Uncertainty, suspicion, deteriorated vendor relationships, and permanently harmed professional reputations are the inevitable byproducts of this scenario.

NEGOTIATION SKILLS

Outside help

Although the professional associations representing North American materiel practitioners have given little attention to the theoretical or practical aspects of negotiation skills, private and public management development organizations have made available a variety of seminars and cassette tapes.[2-5] The most effective training school is experience, but for the new entrant into the health care procurement field or for those unable to acquire the necessary skills through work experience, seminar attendance provides a basic set of understandable precepts, usually supplemented by classroom simulations of actual negotiation sessions.

Staff responsibilities

Health care administrative personnel often feel compelled, because of the increased number of public and semipublic funding mechanisms underwriting health care costs, to proclaim publicly the full details of negotiated contracts to satisfy what are assumed to be the agencies' needs to be satisfied that cost containment has been maximized. Experience suggests that even functioning in a totally government-funded situation, the effective, efficient operation of the institution is the responsibility of the board membership through the senior management staff. The board members must accept the fact that full responsibility rests with the materiel organization to secure the most effective and economic supply arrangements with the freedom to exercise fully, without restrictions, negotiation skills in the pursuit of this goal.

Some boards have had considerable involvement in contract decisions and have reserved the right to handle certain contracts judged to be of particular significance to the financial condition of the institution. Senior administration must convince board members that the staff professionals are completely responsible for all purchased supply and service requirements. With this acceptance of total responsibility, it is then incumbent on the materiel staff members to demonstrate their ability.

The institution should recruit an accomplished purchasing professional from the nonhealth care sector, if the existing staff members demonstrate an inability to develop negotiation talents. Purchasing personnel with intelligence, interest, and dedication to their craft who have not been exposed to theoretical sessions or the example of well-seasoned associates will have, as a normal part of career development, identified opportunities for reducing

costs by price increase restraint, vendor stocking, and inventory reduction clauses in contracts. This occurs even if an overall set of objectives and achievement strategy has not been developed at the prebid stage.

NEGOTIATION STRATEGIES

An essential prerequisite for successful negotiation is provision of a thorough groundwork before the actual negotiation session begins. An extensive bibliography exists, and such specialists as Nierenberg and Zeif are providing training and education through textbooks and seminars.[6] Other texts, particularly those that stress psychological aspects, are of limited value to the person with limited experience, as they could cause the individual to question his or her competence and ability in an area that appears to require formal training as a social scientist or psychologist. Initially, selective reading of basic practical material can be supplemented later by more analytical reading material, which can be more easily related to actual situations.[7-9]

Listing objectives

The groundwork should consist of an exhaustive written listing of the objectives to be attained, and these objectives should be developed by an intelligent and realistic review of the importance of the commodity group or service to the institution in terms of criticality, value of expenditure, volume of usage, capability of the chosen vendor, and pricing strategies of the particular commodity market. For example a roof renovation contract may have a certain completion date as a high priority. The agreement of both parties to a realistic premium-penalty clause may therefore be a significant objective.

In an oligopolistic market situation for a high-volume surgery product with an established "price leader," the negotiation of confidential discounts may be unattainable, but the negotiation of payment deferral for six months after acceptance of goods may be realizable. Depending on prime lending rates this may represent a $7^1/_2$ percent saving, and may lead to further financial benefit for the institution, if the finance department is skilled at maximizing short-term investments. The purchasing negotiator should be involved in contract situations as varied as property and public liability insurance coverage, bulk medical gas supply, patient television service, computerized diagnostic equipment, and needles, syringes, and sutures; no single negotiation objective formula will suit such a wide spectrum of products and services.

Medical and surgical consumable supplies negotiations will probably focus on price increase restraint, volume rebate schedules, guaranteed inventory availability, and stockless, paperless purchasing systems. Equipment purchase negotiations may involve premium-penalty clauses relating to delivery schedules, discounts for additional purchases within an agreed time scale, service responsibilities, and consignment spares inventory within the institution, particularly if inhouse service and maintenance are contemplated.

Remaining flexible

Because the negotiation process is essentially one of proposal and counter-proposal, it is useful to prepare two lists of requirements: a basic minimum set of objectives and a starting list. For example, to achieve a 6-month deferred payment system, the initial request may petition 12-month payment deferral. It is essential for both parties to remain flexible and be able to respond to the unexpected demand or concession. Flexibility may result in achieving greater benefits than had originally been anticipated although in a different form.

There is some mystique associated with the term *negotiation,* but anyone who has purchased a new automobile has some basic understanding of the process. Both parties will have a minimum figure held in reserve for the declaration of the final position. If both buyer and seller are serious and wish to reach agreement, a

---

Anyone who has purchased a new automobile has some basic understanding of the negotiation process.

---

contract will result. Not all negotiation efforts are successful during the first session, but this should not be considered a condemnation of the process. If both parties have time available, an apparent deadlock can be considered as part of the overall negotiation framework. A deadlock permits both sides to reassess their positions and produce new proposals that can result in a final contract of mutual benefit.

The principles of negotiation are applicable whether pursued by an individual institution purchasing representative or by a multihospital group purchasing team, and represent the results of a more mature purchasing profession. The ability to negotiate terms and conditions of an increased financial benefit to the institution enhances the reputation of the materiel-purchasing organization, and will develop the confidence of the senior administrative staff by providing increased opportunities for the materiel-purchasing department to play an enlarged role as part of the senior management team. The development and effective use of negotiation skills will aid in banishing the traditional view of purchasing as a "basement level" clerical function.

REFERENCES

1. Housley, C. "The Prime Supplier Contract: Getting the Most for the Hospital's Supply Dollar." *Hospital Materiel Management Quarterly* 1:3 (February 1980).

2. "Managing Vendors and Supplies." 1-day seminar provided by Business and Professional Research Institute, Princeton, N.J.

3. "Negotiating Leverage" cassette from AMR c/o PHM Services, Ltd., Rexdale, Ontario, Canada.

4. Advanced Management Research Seminar. "Successful Negotiating."

5. Advanced Management Research Seminar. "Strategies, Execution, Pitfalls."

6. "The Art of Negotiating." Seminar sponsored by Nierenberg-Zeif Associates.

7. Caler, H.H. *Winning the Negotiation*. New York: Hawthorn Books (1979).

8. Karrass, C.L. *Give & Take; The Complete Guide to Negotiating Strategies & Tactics* (New York: T.Y. Crowell Co. 1974).

9. Nierenberg, G.I. *Fundamentals of Negotiating*. New York: Hawthorn Books (1973).

Appendix A

Regina General Hospital

Materials Management Department
FOURTEENTH AVENUE & ST. JOHN STREET, REGINA,
SASKATCHEWAN S4P OW5

REQUEST FOR QUOTATION

**Telephone: (306) 522-1811 Ext. 375, 239 or 216
or (306) 523-5588**   Date_____

Your quotation should reach this office by _____
Return one copy of this form regardless of whether you quote.
Prices should be prepaid to Regina General Hospital.
Prices **should not** include Federal Sales Tax.
Prices are subject to Saskatchewan Provincial H & E Tax.
The attached terms and conditions shall be applicable whenever deemed
   appropriate.
All quotations shall provide delivery information.
Absolute confidentiality of commercial information will be observed.

Please find attached a listing of central inventory products from our medical and surgical category showing hospital catalogue number, product description, and average monthly usage data. It is our intention that this product listing will form part of a "Prime Vendor Agreement" after Supplier Proposals, which should include price commitments, are analyzed.

If necessary, in order to fully identify any products in the listing, it will be possible to arrange a specific visit to the hospital by an agreement with the Director of Materials Management or Purchasing Manager, for this purpose. You should not feel restricted when making your proposals as equivalent products will be consid-

ered for any exclusive items, although samples will be required with your submission. It is considered that the essential terms of this proposal are as follows:

1. Agreement may be cancelled by thirty (30) days written notice by either party.

2. Pricing may only be revised semi-annually and shall be on the basis of written evidence of changes to landed costs. Pricing will be established on the basis of established percentages above distributor's base costs.

3. Supplier shall maintain a 60-day inventory of items covered by the agreement at the nearest distribution

center to Regina and shall be prepared to accept random inventory checks without prior notification.

4. A paperless release system shall be used for "calling-off" supplies and delivery shall occur within a pre-determined time frame with a minimum of 90 percent of the ordered items being received. Failure to achieve the required performance will result in the application of a prescribed penalty formula.

5. An incentive rebate structure will be established based on certain plateaux of dollar volume.

6. The final terms and conditions of any contract ensuing from this enquiry shall be subject to negotiation by both parties involved.

Signature of Company Representative

Date

Materials Management Department
Regina General Hospital

Appendix B
Regina General Hospital

Terms and Conditions

1. The Contract is between _____ (hereafter called the Supplier) and the Regina General Hospital (hereafter called the Buyer).
2. The Contract may be terminated by either party upon delivery of written notice, at least thirty (30) days prior to the desired date of termination.
3. The Buyer shall, for the term of this Contract, purchase all requirements from the Supplier, provided that such items are immediately available.
4. Except in the case of prior notice of nonavailability if the Supplier cannot supply total requirements the Buyer shall have the right to purchase the balance elsewhere and *debit the Supplier any price variation so incurred.*
5. If Buyer's requirements change materially altering the Supplier's costs, either party may, in writing, request negotiation of contract prices.
6. Written request for a price increase must be presented to the Materials Management Department of the Regina General Hospital thirty (30) days in advance of the effective date of the price increase providing details to substantiate the increase such as copies of manufacturer's price increase notification letters. The Buyer may reject the price increase and terminate the Contract by written notice to the Supplier (as allowed for in Paragraph 1) prior to the stated effective date of the price increase.
7. The Supplier also has the responsibility to submit in writing notification of price decreases to the Buyer and to pass the benefits of all general price decreases on to the Buyer.
8. No substitution of material shall be permitted on product to be supplied unless previously agreed to by the Buyer and the acceptance confirmed in writing.
9. Upon expiry of this contract, if renewal does not occur, the Buyer agrees to accept liability for stocks held by the Supplier within the terms of this contract subject to the condition that there will be no liability for items normally stocked by the Supplier as general inventory.
10. The terms and conditions detailed above are subject to further negotiation, if necessary.

Appendix C
Extract from Regina General Hospital

TENDERING GUIDELINES—MARCH 1975

Preparation of tender requests

The request is developed on a quotation request form which details the entire specifications of the equipment or supplies being tendered. Details of any special requirements required will be indicated on this form, such as a systems contract situation, guaranteed 24-hour delivery, and firm pricing for a specific period of time. In the case of contract tender requests a copy of the recently instituted terms and conditions requirements are included with the tender request.

Potential supplier selection

This phase is of critical importance and follows immediately the completion of the tender request. It is essential that selection is made in a totally impartial manner without favoritism or prejudice and with the objective of including all known, able companies represented in the product market concerned. Selection is currently made on the basis of ability to supply, past performance, existence of local office and warehouse arrangements, and any other particular factors that may apply to specific products. In the medical and surgical equipment field a considerable volume of products are single source items because of exclusive regional distributor arrangements but this is seldom true of the general consumable suppliers. Supplier selection for quotation purposes is still dependent to some extent on acquired knowledge of supplier behavior from experience. It is intended during the course of 1975 to develop a more scientific system of Vendor Analysis based on a points rating system for a set number of factors such as delivery dates achieved, quality, firm price maintenance, and other appropriate factors.

Tender analysis

At the appointed time set for quotation opening, all proposals received are examined. The results are not considered public knowledge unless tender requests have been publicly requested.

An analysis is prepared using the Bid Summary Form. If all conditions are equal the Regina-based company is selected; if this is not possible, Saskatchewan-based enterprises are chosen in preference to those based elsewhere. Further negotiations may occur with the company selected to be the supplier to determine a number of commercial objectives. A primary objective is to minimize hospital investment in inventory but certain guarantees of supplier's Regina stock levels are required, according to the importance of the product involved. The principal criteria are total value offered by the supply source which is a combination of pricing and the values achieved by reduced hospital inventories contributed by local supplier stocking and other negotiated benefits.

Avoiding conflict-of-interest and related organization problems

Michael K. Gire
Attorney
Bricker & Eckler
Columbus, Ohio

CONFLICT OF INTEREST

Definition

ALTHOUGH the term *conflict of interest* is often associated with some form of financial misconduct, its legal meaning encompasses a much larger universe of prohibited behavior. The legal definition of conflict of interest is generally considered to be any situation in which regard for one legal duty tends to lead to a disregard of another legal duty. It is, then, any situation wherein a person acting in a fiduciary capacity in relation to a hospital has a competing interest or duality of interest that may cause that person to act in other than the best interest of the hospital. Conflict of interest may exist regardless of whether this person stands to make a personal gain.

A classic example of how conflict-of-interest problems can be present in hospitals occurred in the case of *Stern* v. *Lucy Webb Hayes National Training School for*

Deaconesses and Missionaries.[1] In the *Stern* case, several members of the board of trustees of Sibley Hospital in Washington, D.C. were connected with local financial institutions. Over a period of several years, liquid assets of the hospital were kept in accounts at these financial institutions that drew inadequate or no interest. Patients of Sibley Hospital, as purchasers of health services from the hospital, filed a class action suit against five of the trustees, the financial institutions, and the hospital alleging that the defendant trustees had conspired to enrich themselves and the financial institutions by favoring those institutions in financial dealings with the hospital.

Following a trial on the issues raised by the plaintiffs, the United States District Court for the District of Columbia issued a decision that there was no evidence that a conspiracy existed among the defendant trustees. The judge was, however, critical of the self-dealing that took place between the trustees and the financial institutions with which they were affiliated. The judge indicated that a trustee of a charitable hospital should always avoid active participation in a transaction in which the trustee or a corporation with which the trustee is associated has a significant intent. The court held that a person acting in a fiduciary capacity in the governing of a hospital's affairs has a continuing duty of loyalty and care in the management of the hospital's fiscal and investment affairs, and acts in violation of that duty if:

1. The person fails, while assigned to a particular committee of the board having stated financial or investment responsibilities under the bylaws of the corporation, to use diligence in supervising and periodically inquiring into the actions of those officers, employees, and outside experts to whom any duty to make day-to-day financial or investment decisions within such committee's responsibility has been assigned or delegated;

2. The person knowingly permits the hospital to enter into a business transaction with himself or herself or with any corporation, partnership, or association in which he or she holds a position as trustee, director, partner, general manager, principal officer, or substantial shareholder without previously having informed all persons charged with approving that transaction of his or her interest or position and of any significant facts known to him or her indicating that the transaction might not be in the best interests of the hospital;

3. The person actively participates in, except as required by the preceding paragraph, or votes in favor of a decision by the board or any committee or subcommittee thereof to transact business with himself or herself or with any corporation, partnership, or association in which he or she holds a position as trustee, director, partner, general manager, principal officer, or substantial shareholder; or

4. The person fails to perform his or her duties honestly, in good faith, and with reasonable diligence and care.[2]

While the *Stern* case demonstrates how a conflict-of-interest situation can arise with the trustees of a hospital, its principles are also applicable to officers and employees of a hospital in making financial and procurement decisions.

Avoiding conflict of interest

The importance of the *Stern* case is its enunciation of the two key elements that should be emphasized to avoid conflict-of-interest problems:

1. Putting into place a mechanism whereby there can be full disclosure of conflicts of interest and any material facts to ensure that all actions are taken in the best interest of the hospital; and

2. That a person abstain from any active participation on behalf of the hospital in any transaction when the person has a conflict of interest.

The preferred method for avoiding conflict-of-interest problems in a hospital is to establish written conflict-of-interest policies.

The preferred method for avoiding conflict-of-interest problems in a hospital is to establish written conflict-of-interest policies. The purpose of these policies is to address the key elements identified in the *Stern* case: (1) disclosure of potential conflicts of interest; and (2) procedures to be followed when a conflict of interest exists. The Joint Commission on the Accreditation of Hospitals (JCAH) now requires in Standard III for the Governing Body that just such a policy must be adopted: "The governing body shall have a written conflict-of-interest policy that addresses disclosure and guidelines for resolutions."[3] It is interesting to note, however, that in a recent survey by the American Hospital Association (AHA) of hospital governing boards, only 25.1 percent of the hospitals responding indicated that governing body members were required to file written declarations of potential conflicts of interest.[4]

Disclosure

The purpose of a written policy that requires disclosure of potential conflicts of interest is to ensure that all potential situations in which a duality of interest may be present are fully known to persons acting in a decision-making capacity. Generally, hospitals that have adopted such disclosure requirements have limited coverage to members of the hospital's board of trustees or board of directors. To be effective at avoiding conflicts of interest at all levels of hospital management, however, consideration should be given to expanding the disclosure requirements to include officers and employees handling procurement and financial matters for the hospital where potential conflicts of interest may arise.

The specific matters that should be included under a written disclosure policy must be determined by each hospital individually. General areas of disclosure that should be considered include the following:

1. Any positions or financial interests held in any concern from which the hospital purchases goods or services;

2. Any positions or financial interests held in any concern that is in competition with the hospital;

3. Any direct or indirect competition with the hospital in the purchase or sale of property or property rights, interest, or services;

4. Any governing body memberships or managerial or consultative relations

with any outside concern that does business with or competes with the hospital;

5. Any gifts, excessive entertainment, or funds received from any outside concern that either provides goods or services to the hospital, seeks to provide goods or services to the hospital, does business with the hospital, or is in competition with the hospital;

6. Any disclosure or use of information relating to the hospital for the personal profit of the individual or to the advantage of any business entity in which the individual holds a position or has a financial interest; and

7. Any other matter in which the individual's ability to act in the best interest of the hospital may be compromised by a competing interest outside the hospital.

The written conflict-of-interest statements should be filed on a regular basis (e.g., annually), and reviewed by persons designated for that purpose. Written disclosure statements filed by members of the hospital's board and officers, could, for example, be reviewed and kept on file with a committee of the board designated for that purpose. Written disclosure statements filed by certain specified employees could, for example, be reviewed and kept on file with the officer of the hospital who is in charge of those employees.

In addition to the written conflict-of-interest disclosure statements, at any time that a conflict of interest actually arises, the person having the conflict of interest should again make disclosure of such a conflict, and that disclosure should be documented (e.g., in the minutes of the board).

Handling a conflict of interest

A hospital's conflict-of-interest policy should also set forth what policies to follow in the event that a conflict of interest occurs. With respect to boards of trustees or boards of directors, the corporation law of the state in which the hospital is located will very often govern how conflicts of interest should be resolved. Therefore, hospital counsel should be consulted to determine state law requirements. General items to be addressed include the following:

1. Whether the board member can vote or use his or her influence in any matter in which the board member may have a conflict of interest;

2. Whether the board member can be counted for quorum purposes on any matter in which the board member has a conflict of interest;

3. Whether the board member is permitted to briefly state his or her views or respond to questions relating to a matter in which the board member has a conflict of interest; and

4. Whether approval must be given by a majority (or more) of the disinterested board members in a matter in which a board member has a conflict of interest.

If state law does not address the problem of officers and employees, the governing board will have to determine the policies to follow when an officer or employee has a conflict of interest. General policies that might be considered include the following:

1. To whom the officer or employee should report the conflict of interest;
2. Whether the officer or employee will be permitted to participate in any transactions on behalf of the hospital in which the officer or employee has a conflict of interest;
3. What the role of an officer or employee should be in any instance where such officer or employee has a conflict of interest; and
4. Who should have authority to act on behalf of an officer or employee who has a conflict of interest.

It must be emphasized that a hospital is not necessarily precluded from entering into financial or business transactions with a person or business entity when a conflict of interest is present. So long as proper disclosure has been made and the hospital's policies governing how the affairs of the hospital are to be managed in conflict-of-interest situations are followed, the transaction is not, *per se,* impermissible. But, in the absence of clear policies relating to disclosure requirements and the handling of conflict-of-interest situations, hospital governing boards may not only find that the hospital is not in compliance with the JCAH standards, but they may also find themselves faced with litigation similar to the *Stern* case.

RELATED ORGANIZATIONS

Although a hospital is not necessarily precluded from entering into transactions where one or more persons associated with it have a conflict of interest, care must be taken to ensure that the hospital does not jeopardize a portion of its Medicare reim- bursement by dealing with related organizations.

Regulations

Under the regulations of the Department of Health and Human Services (HHS)[5] and Chapter X of the *Medicare Provider Reimbursement Manual,*[6] special rules apply to reimbursement for hospital costs applicable to services, facilities, and supplies furnished to the hospital by organizations related to the hospital by common ownership or control. If a hospital does purchase (or lease) services, facilities, or supplies from a related organization, the allowable cost of the hospital is limited to the actual costs to the related organization, regardless of the price paid by the hospital.

The "definitions" sections of the HHS regulations and the *Medicare Provider Reimbursement Manual* indicate that:

- "Related to the provider" means that the provider to a significant extent is associated or affiliated with, or has control of or is controlled by the organization furnishing the services, facilities, or supplies;
- "Common ownership" exists when an individual or individuals possess significant ownership or equity in the provider and the institution or organization servicing the provider; and
- "Control" exists where an individual or an organization has the power, directly or indirectly, to significantly influence or direct the actions or policies of an organization or institution.

The tests for determining common ownership and common control are applied separately. If common ownership

*For nonprofit organizations, owner-
ship or equity interest is determined
by reference to the interest in the assets of the organization.*

or common control is present, then the
hospital and the organization are related.

For purposes of determining common
control, the *Medicare Provider Reimbursement Manual* indicates that the facts and
circumstances of each case must be
reviewed to determine whether an individual or individuals possess significant
ownership or equity interest in the hospital
and the supplying organization so as to
make the two entities related by common
ownership. The organizations involved
include sole proprietorships, partnerships,
corporations, trusts or estates, or any other
form of business organization, proprietary
or nonprofit. For nonprofit organizations,
ownership or equity interest is determined
by reference to the interest in the assets of
the organization.[7]

In the examples of common ownership
given in the manual, it is clear that if an
individual has majority ownership of both
a hospital and a supplying organization,
the two entities will be treated as related
organizations. If an individual has less than
majority interest in either the hospital or
the supplying organization, or both, then it
becomes a factual question when significant ownership or equity intent exists.[8]

Examples

For purposes of determining control,
the manual indicates that any kind of

control, whether or not it is legally
enforceable and however it is exercisable
or exercised, must be considered. The
presence of control is determined by
reviewing the facts and circumstances of
each case to ascertain if legal or effective
control exists.[9] The manual gives the
following examples of control:

Example One:

Dr. A is the medical director of a provider,
but he does not have an ownership interest in
the provider. He is also the president and
owner of a supplier organization that provides
various therapeutic services primarily to the
provider. Under the circumstances described,
it will be presumed that Dr. A has the power
to influence or direct both the provider and
the supplying organization, and that the organizations are related to each other by common
control.

Example Two:

Mr. A owns a 60 percent interest in the
provider organization. Mr. A's two sons and
wife together own a 100 percent interest in the
organization supplying the provider. Under the
circumstances described, it will be presumed
that Mr. A has the power to influence and
direct the actions of his family relating to the
operations of the supplying organization, and
that the organizations are related by common
control.

Example Three:

A construction company builds a facility
and leases it to an operating company that
becomes a provider. Mr. A owns a 100 percent
interest in the construction company and a 35
percent interest in the operating company. Mr.
B, a key employee of the construction company, owns a 20 percent interest in the operating
company. Under the circumstances described,
it will be presumed that Mr. A, as the

employer of Mr. B in the construction company, can influence Mr. B's decisions relative to the operation of the provider and that the construction company and the provider are related by common control. (Mr. B would probably not jeopardize his position in the construction company by opposing Mr. A's wishes in the management of the provider.)

Example Four:

Mr. H owns a 45 percent interest in Corporation X, the provider organization. The remaining 55 percent interest is owned by Corporation Y, the supplying organization. Mr. H owns a 100 percent interest in Corporation Y. Mr. H controls 10 percent of Corporation X, his own 45 percent direct interest in Corporation X, and the indirect 55 percent interest owned by Corporation Y. Mr. H has complete control over both the provider and supplying organization; therefore, the organizations are related by control.[10]

While the examples given primarily address proprietary hospitals, it is clear that the control rules also apply to nonprofit hospitals. In Provider Reimbursement Review Board Decision No. 77-D11, a nonprofit hospital that had leased its facilities decided to purchase the hospital building, land, certain equipment, and a clinic from a for-profit real estate corporation. Four of the shareholders of the real estate corporation, owning 80 percent of the stock in the aggregate, were physicians who were also on the nine-member board of trustees of the nonprofit hospital. One of the four physicians served on the executive committee, and another was the medical director for the hospital. The hospital reported depreciation expense for the facilities purchased based on the purchase price paid to the real estate corporation.

The intermediary limited the hospital's basis for depreciation to the basis of the real estate corporation because it concluded that the hospital and the real estate corporation were related entities. The Provider Reimbursement Review Board concurred with the intermediary because it found that the stockholders of the real estate corporation were in a position and had the ability to control or significantly influence the actions of the nonprofit hospital[11]:

. . . indisputable evidence clearly showed that there existed the ability to control or influence, directly or indirectly, the actions or policies of the institution.[12]

Due to the related-organization rules concerning reimbursement, hospital dealings with organizations owned or controlled by persons in a position to control or significantly influence the hospital must be given close scrutiny. The written conflict-of-interest disclosure statements can be of assistance in avoiding related-organization problems by alerting the hospital to situations that may bring the related-organization rules into play.

As a matter of procedure, and to conform to JCAH requirements, hospitals should adopt conflict-of-interest policies that require disclosure of potential conflicts of interest, and that provide guidelines for action in the event that a conflict of interest should occur. The hospital's conflict-of-interest policy should be coordinated with the purchase of services, facilities, and supplies to ensure that the hospital does not enter into transactions with related organizations that could result in adverse reimbursement consequences.

REFERENCES

1. Stern v. Lucy Webb Hayes National Training School for Deaconesses and Missionaries, Inc., 381 F. Supp. 1003 (D.D.C. 1974).
2. Ibid.
3. Joint Commission on the Accreditation of Hospitals. *Accreditation Manual for Hospitals* (Chicago: JCAH 1981) p. 52.
4. Nigosian, G. "Board Operating Practices Subject of AHA Survey." *Hospitals, JAHA* 54:22 (November 1980) p. 81.
5. 42 C.F.R. §405.427 (1980).
6. U.S. Department of Health and Human Services. *Medicare Provider Reimbursement Manual*, HIM 15-1 (Washington, D.C.: Health Care Financing Administration 1980).
7. Ibid. 1004.1, p. 3–10.
8. Ibid. 1004.3, p. 3–10.
9. Ibid.
10. Ibid. 1004.4, p. 4–10.
11. Commerce Clearing House. *Medicare and Medicaid Guides* Transfer Binder ¶28, 301-28, 800 (Chicago: CCH 1977) p. 9386.
12. Ibid. p. 9391.

Approved products lists are imperative to effective purchasing

George Y. Hersch
Assistant Director
Materiel Management
Saint Anthony Hospital
Columbus, Ohio

WITHOUT THE PROPER CONTROLS, materiel management might soon be on a course of self-destruction. With thousands of supplies already in the hospital system, and thousands more trying to find their way in, how can the hospital ensure that only acceptable products are being used? One important control readily available to the materiel manager is the approved products list.

An approved products list is a written documentation of supplies approved for use in a particular hospital. Such lists control the acquisition of medical and surgical supplies and guide the various departments in materiel ordering, two highly important functions in the hospital's supply complex.

Suppose that Dr. X likes Pharmaseal exam gloves, Dr. Y likes Tomac exam gloves, and Dr. Z likes Parke Davis exam gloves. Can a hospital ever hope to achieve any economies of scale by permitting all three types of exam gloves in its institution? Can it ensure that there will not be excessive inventory to satisfy all three preferences? Keeping track of thousands of other products with two or more manufacturers could get dangerously out of control. However with an approved products list, the type of exam glove for general use in the hospital would already be identified as available through a preselected vendor and purchased at an established price.

Besides eliminating abusive personal product preference, the approved products list offers another type of control. If alphabetized by manufacturer then further categorized by department, it offers a guide that will help the departments maintain ordering consistency. So while there may be a turnover in personnel responsible for requisitioning, the approved products list is a legacy to the next person made responsible for ordering supplies.

HAVING A GAME PLAN

With so many thousands of supplies in a hospital, how does a materiel manager begin the arduous task of listing them all? Obviously it is important to have a good game plan. The materiel manager who has taken inventories already has a good start. These records will readily furnish a good accounting of which products are in use. If such records are not available, the materiel manager may wish to begin listing supplies from requisitions that pass through his or her department. This is most effective when the hospital is totally committed to centralized purchasing.

Departmental emphasis

At best, either of these two methods is just a beginning to the development of a good approved products list. The main thrust should come from the departments themselves. For it is here that the most comprehensive development of the approved products list occurs. Once it is explained to department heads how vital the approved products list is for cost containment and materiel control, cooperation should begin. Materiel managers should not be discouraged, however, if the departments are not enthusiastic about the approved products list. Developing these lists is a time-consuming chore.

It is helpful to distribute a core listing of supplies to each department based on either inventory listings or data gathered from supply requisitions. If a start has already been provided, the task of completing the approved products lists will be viewed as being easier.

It should be emphasized that this is a project designed to aid both materiel management and other departments. In essence, the materiel manager is sanctioning supplies being used in the hospital. It should be made clear that after the approved products list is developed, all new supplies coming into the hospital must first be approved by the Evaluation and Standardization of Products (ESP) committee. The sanctioning opportunity should encourage the departments to be comprehensive.

Flexibility and clarity

Because other departments are being asked to cooperate with materiel management in assuming a large portion of the work, it is important to establish reasonable completion dates. It may take some departments, like surgery, several months to generate such a list; others, such as occupational therapy, may be able to complete the list in a few days. If extensions are requested, the materiel manager should be willing to grant them. The goal is to get good information that will help all departments. However, no more than three months should probably be allowed to complete the project.

The materiel manager should be clear about the types of items to be included in the list. They should be disposable items ordered every two weeks or sooner. This includes a myriad of supplies, such as medical gasses, plastic linen bags and trash can liners, office supplies, dietary paper goods, and food staples. While a two-week turn of inventory is considered good, it may be advisable to make a rule that the maximum reorder quantity not exceed a month without special permission. This will build in flexibility for some supplies where the minimum order cannot be used up in a month. In any case it is important to emphasize that orders exceeding a month's supply require special permission and justification.

DEVELOPING A FORMAT

What to include

To be comprehensive the list should include the following information: name of the department, manufacturer, vendor, product, catalog number, product description, packaging information (i.e., how many per box), two-week quantity, and cost of the item. Each page should have the same format and be dedicated to a single manufacturer. For example Pharmaseal may head the page with a listing of all Pharmaseal items purchased for a particular department within the hospital.

The list might include surgeon's gloves, connecting tubing, stopcocks, catheter plugs, etc. When such a list is developed by manufacturer, it affords materiel management the opportunity to adjust easily the prices of all supplies purchased from a particular manufacturer should a new price list be issued. It also tells at a glance how many items are purchased from a manufacturer. This is also helpful when a competitive manufacturer requests information on the types of products purchased. At a glance, the amount of potential business can be relayed by quoting the types of products and estimated annual quantities per product. With this information readily available, it is possible to save thousands of dollars on one product alone.

Like chapters in a text, each department's approved products list will meld together into a large approved products book. And just as the number of pages in a chapter vary, so will the number of manufacturers in each department vary. Larger supply-consuming departments will have more manufacturers on their list. For instance anesthesiology may list ten manufacturers; surgery may list 50 or more manufacturers.

The breakdown

Developing an approved products book by department also has certain advantages. To control the number of requisitions that flow through the materiel management department, there must be a policy of assigning each department a specific ordering day. This will accomplish two objectives. It will provide an even flow of requisitions to the buyer. By doing this the ordering will be spread out evenly during the week. A smoother flow of requisitions will have a better effect on the receiving department. Effective scheduling of ordering can eliminate major deliveries arriving at the same time and slowing the receiving function. Of course since there are only five working days in a week, several departments may be required to order on the same day. Thus it is advisable to combine departments that have supply requirements from the same vendor. By departmentalizing the approved products book, the buyer will have to skim through fewer product lists to obtain pricing information that must be applied to the requisition before it is converted to a purchase order complete with item pricing, approved vendor, an approved signature, and a purchase order number.

The other alternative is to arrange the approved products book alphabetically by manufacturer. This makes it easier to update those twice-a-year price changes, but more difficult for the buyer to thumb through hundreds of manufacturers on a daily basis to get pricing for each department. Thus at the expense of some redundancy in listing the same item more than once, further subdividing the approved products book by department seems to be expedient in the long run.

MAKING THE LIST WORK

Once all this information has been assimilated from the departments, the materiel manager will have—probably for the first time—a global view of the hospital supply situation. As materiel managers become acquainted with these lists, they may begin to notice some duplication in the supply line. Why for instance does the emergency room have *x* catheter and the nursing units have *y* catheter? Chances are that neither of the two areas realizes what the other area is using. And possibly neither area has a strong preference. This provides a prime opportunity to standardize. This decision should be made by the ESP committee. Before a decision on standardizing is reached, however, each area should have a chance to present its case before the committee. Although the ESP committee should have the ultimate authority on deciding what will be the approved supply in the hospital, its role is to assist the hospital in its cost-containment efforts while maximizing the highest quality of patient care. The committee should not create hard feelings and should at all times offer impartial judgments.

Negotiations and surveys

The approved products book will also help with vendor negotiations. Because the products are already listed by manufacturer, it becomes easy to negotiate an entire line of a particular manufacturer's items. Also, because two-week quantities are already listed, projections on annualized quantities can be made for each product. In fact the list can become an automatic bid sheet by blanking out the prices and

The ESP committee's role is to assist the hospital in cost-containment efforts. The committee should not create hard feelings and should at all times offer impartial judgments.

giving copies of the sheet to vendors offering the same manufacturer's line of items. The vendor can fill in the prices and the materiel manager can choose the vendor that offers these products at the best price.

One note of caution, however. Each vendor in the bid process should agree in writing to a specific amount of time under which these items will be price protected. Taking that one step further, the materiel manager may also wish to have vendors agree to a maximum percentage of price increase at the end of this time period.

The approved products book can also be used in completing price surveys initiated by group purchasing, third party payers, or the hospital. These surveys often ask for information pertaining to the manufacturer, vendor, complete description, catalog number, annual usage, and price of a supply item. With such information already tabulated, all the materiel manager need do is look it up.

Checklists

These lists can also aid in checking for product recalls. If a recall letter is received about a particular product from a manufacturer or if a recall notice appears in a publication such as *Health Devices Alerts*, materiel management can immediately identify whether the hospital uses the

_____ No Recalls This Month

_____ Recall(s) This Month

Manufacturer: _____

Item: _____

Reason for Recall: _____

_____

_____

Date Materiel Management Notified: _____

Department(s) Notified	Individuals	Date
_____	_____	_____
_____	_____	_____
_____	_____	_____

Action Taken for Recalled Item: _____

_____

_____

_____

Figure 1. Sample department of materiel management recall report.

Department: _____   Inventory Date: _____

Manufacturer-Vendor _____   Participants: _____

Page _____ of _____

	Approved Product	Information				Inventory Information		
Catalog #	Description	Qty	Ut.	2-wk. Qty.	Cost/Ut.	Qty.	Ut.	Total ($)

Figure 2. Sample approved products/inventory list.

product and, if so, what departments stock it. Should any products be affected by the recall, all that needs to be done is to check with the using departments to see if they have any of the product lot numbers being recalled. This action should be reported to the administrator in a monthly recall report. (See Figure 1.)

Finally the list can be used to take inventory. If adapted with a count column and a price extension column, it can become a valuable checklist and record for annual, semiannual, or quarterly inventories. (See Figure 2.)

Special categories

Because an approved product may be back ordered from a vendor for numerous reasons, the materiel manager may wish to have an addendum to the approved products book on approved substitutions. Product substitutions may be objectionable, so they should be examined by the ESP committee after a supply "crisis" has passed. Just as any new product coming into the hospital should have ESP approval, so should product substitutes. If the committee finds the substitute unsuitable, the materiel manager should find another one that provides a better temporary replacement for the next crisis. Once the committee approves that, it can be added to the approved products substitutes list. Eventually nearly every product should have an approved substitute counterpart. So when the next crisis arises, all that need be done is cross-reference the product in the approved products book and the problem is abated. Most important, a policy on

substitutes must be developed. (See Appendix.)

Although approved products lists can be developed for every department, there are some areas where they definitely are not appropriate. Such areas include equipment parts, miscellaneous office supplies, and prostheses. While it may seem obvious that these kinds of materials cannot be standardized, it is equally important to realize that every system must have a certain amount of built-in flexibility or it loses credibility.

PLANNING FOR EMERGENCIES

If an emergency arises that violates the approved products list, there should be a plan of action to deal with it. Suppose that during the first day in the operating room, a newly appointed staff physician has an allergic reaction to the surgeon's gloves that have long been approved for use in the institution. Materiel management can get approval from administration to honor the request for purchasing another type of glove and justify the action at the next ESP committee meeting. It could be that the committee will approve the glove only for this physician. At any rate, a small crisis has been averted, an intelligent decision reached, and the system maintains credibility.

Developing a comprehensive approved products list takes a great deal of time and effort. Once the list begins to work, however, hospital staff will question how they ever functioned without it.

Appendix
Department of Materiel Management

St. Anthony Hospital
Columbus, Ohio

Subject: *Product Substitution*

Objective: To assure that the desired quality of supplies is attained in the purchasing process.

Policy Statement: It shall be the policy of the Department of Materiel Management that no product substitutions on behalf of the supplier will be allowable.

Procedural Documentation: Products may not be substituted in any manner by the supplier, and any such substitutions shall be returned to the supplier at the supplier's expense.

The Materiel Manager may make substitution if an item is unavailable from supplier and stock is sufficiently low to warrant substitution.

In making such a substitution, the Materiel Manager must check the Approved Substitute Products List and acquire only substitute products on that list.

If the unavailable item does not have an approved substitute, the Materiel Manager should contact supervisors of the using areas to determine what an acceptable substitute should be. The item should be of equitable quality to the ESP approved item.

Once the acceptable substitute is determined, the Materiel Manager should take this product to the next regularly scheduled ESP committee meeting for formal approval.

Purchase on your terms, not theirs

Dennis C. Kaldor
Director
Material Management
Kenosha Memorial Hospital
Kenosha, Wisconsin

TOO OFTEN in the hospital purchase process materiel managers openly and carelessly accept whatever terms of sale the vendor states. Materiel managers accept vendors' policies and terms and do not challenge the conditions of sale. They also accept the price, charges for shipping, discount schedule, and credit terms, as well as such other "soft" dictates as back orders, delays in shipment, misshipment, inflated orders, and product substitution.

If a hospital has no policies as part of a purchase contract then it is literally at the mercy of the supplier. It is important for hospitals to be as aggressive in the purchase process as their counterparts in industry. Availability of medical equipment and supplies is certainly as important to a hospital as availability of engine parts is to an auto manufacturer. When vendors accept orders for supplies, they must recognize the importance of providing those supplies as promised or face the risk of penalty.

In April 1979 Kenosha Memorial Hospital began to implement the process of centralized purchasing. Each department previously had ordered its own equipment and supplies, and only capital expenditures went through any kind of central purchasing process. It was apparent that there was little control in the purchases being made and virtually no control over vendor policies and terms of sale.

In instituting centralized purchasing, the hospital wanted to purchase from an advantageous position whenever possible. It was felt that all terms of the sale should be negotiable, not just the price of the item involved. Each vendor who had received a check from the hospital during the past fiscal year was sent a letter announcing the new purchasing department and the procedures to be followed.

With these procedures established as general policies, materiel management was in a position to deal objectively with vendors in establishing conditions of purchase and sale. It was recognized that several of the points would be in conflict with vendor policies and procedures. On some subjects materiel management held firm. On others it was willing to compromise. Any concessions from these policies, however, were specifically negotiated with individual suppliers.

To add strength to hospital policies and to reinforce them, as daily orders were placed, the major points were included on the printed purchase. (Vendors were to accept these conditions as a contractual obligation.) These points, printed on the reverse side of the purchase order, were subject to negotiation. If deviations or omissions were to be allowed, they were so noted and initialed on the purchase order. The points as they are printed on the purchase order appear in the Appendix.

Through aggressive purchasing the hospital stands to gain in several areas. These rewards are realized in hard cash as well as intangible benefits. In controlling the terms of purchase the entire materiel management function of the hospital benefits—from point of purchase to more reliable availability of supplies in all departments.

Appendix
Terms and conditions of purchase

Acceptance. This order is for the purchase and sale of the goods (herein referred to as "the Articles") and/or services described on the front hereof and is Buyer's offer to Seller. Acknowledgment hereof by Seller to Buyer shall constitute Seller's acceptance of such order, including all of the terms and conditions herein set out. In the absence of such acknowledgment, commencement of delivery of the Articles and/or services and acceptance of such deliveries by Buyer shall constitute a firm contract on the terms and conditions hereof.

This order is subject to the following terms and conditions and no others unless there is a signed overriding agreement between the parties prepared by Buyer. No purchase order is valid without the signature of the purchasing agent or director of materiel management. A qualified representative of the supplier or manufacturer is required to provide the necessary inservice support to all the appropriate hospital personnel.

Packing. The Articles shall be packed and shipped by Seller in accordance with Buyer's instructions and good commercial practice and so as to ensure that no damage shall result from weather or transportation. No goods or services shall be received, nor invoice paid, unless there is a valid purchase order for those goods or services prior to delivery. Purchase order number must appear on invoices and shipping containers of all shipments.

Warranty—Product. Seller warrants that all the Articles will be free from defects in material and workmanship and, if ordered for a stated purpose, will be fit for such purpose. The equipment or product must pass inspection for safety, performance, and compliance with manufacturer's specifications prior to acceptance for clinical use. It must be provided with a minimum of three complete user manuals, which will include instructions for use, warnings of potential hazards, parts lists, schematics, and service and maintenance requirements, where applicable. The warranty shall begin on the date that incoming inspection is passed.

Payment to Vendor will not be authorized until these conditions are fulfilled. Seller also warrants that to the extent the Articles are not manufactured pursuant to detailed designs furnished by Buyer, they will be free from defects in design. Such warranties, including warranties prescribed by law, shall run a Buyer, its successors, assigns, and customers, and to user of the Articles, for a period of one year after delivery or such longer period as may be prescribed by law or additional agreement.

The equipment or product must pass inspection for safety, performance, and compliance with manufacturer's specifications prior to acceptance for clinical use.

All equipment must carry at least a one-year warranty on parts and labor.

Warranty—Price. Seller warrants that the prices charged Buyer, as indicated on the front side hereof, are no higher than prices charged on orders placed by others for similar quantities on similar conditions subsequent to the last general announced price change. In the event Seller breaches this warranty, the prices of the Articles shall be reduced accordingly retroactively to date of such breach. Price increases unacceptable without notice and acceptance prior to shipment.

Patent Infringement Indemnity. Seller warrants and agrees to defend, indemnify, and hold harmless Buyer, its successors, assigns, customers, and users of Seller's products from and against any claim, loss, damage, or expense arising out of any infringement or claim of infringement of any letters patent, trade name, trademark, copyright, or trade secrets by reason of the sale or use of any Articles purchased hereunder. Buyer shall promptly notify Seller of any such claim.

Buyer-Furnished Property. Seller shall not use, reproduce, or appropriate for, or disclose to, anyone other than Buyer any material, tooling, dies, drawings, designs, and other property or data furnished by Buyer, nor shall Seller use that same to produce or manufacture more Articles than are required hereunder. Title thereto shall remain in Buyer at all times. Seller shall bear the risk of loss or damage to such property furnished by Buyer unless such loss or damage is solely, directly, and proximately caused by Buyer's negligence. All such Buyer-furnished property, together with spoiled and surplus materials, shall be returned to Buyer at termination or completion of this order unless Buyer shall otherwise direct.

Termination. Buyer may cancel this order, in whole or in part, without liability to Buyer, if deliveries are not made at the time and in the quantities specified or in the event of a breach or failure of any of the other terms or conditions hereof.

Buyer may terminate this order in whole or part, at any time for its convenience, by notice to Seller in writing. On receipt by Seller of such notice, Seller shall, and to the extent specified therein, stop work hereunder and the placement of subcontracts, terminate work under subcontracts outstanding hereunder, and take any necessary action to protect property in Seller's possession in which Buyer has or may acquire an interest. Any termination claim must be submitted to Buyer within sixty (60) days after the effective date of the termination.

Any cancellation or termination by Buyer, whether for default or otherwise, shall be without prejudice to any claims for damages or other rights of Buyer against Seller. Buyer shall have the right to audit all elements of any termination claim, and Seller shall make available to Buyer on request all books, records, and papers relating thereto.

Changes. Buyer at any time may make changes in the quantities ordered or in the specifications or drawings relating to the Articles or may change or amend any other term or condition of this order, in which event an equitable adjustment will be made to any price, time of performance, and/or other provisions of this order required to be changed thereby. Any claim for such an adjustment must be made within fifteen (15) days from the date of receipt by Seller of such change.

Compliance with Laws. In filing this order, Seller shall comply with all applicable federal, state, and local laws, and governmental regulations and orders. Seller specifically warrants and guarantees to Buyer:

A . that the Articles are in compliance with Sections 5 and 12 of the Federal Trade Commission Act, and are properly labeled as to content as required by applicable Federal Trade Commission Trade Practice Rules;

B . that the Articles are in compliance with the provisions of the Fair Packaging and Labeling Act;

C . that the Articles are not adulterated or misbranded within the meaning of the Federal Food, Drug, and Cosmetic Act, as amended, or within the meaning of any applicable state or municipal law in which the definitions of adulteration and misbranding are substantially identical with those contained in the Federal Food, Drug, and Cosmetic Act, or are not Articles that may not under the provisions of Sections 404 or 405 of said Act be introduced into interstate commerce or that may not under substantially similar provisions of any state or municipal law be introduced into commerce;

D . that the Articles are in compliance with the Consumer Product Safety Act of 1972;

E . that the Articles are in compliance with the Federal Insecticide, Fungicide, and Rodenticide Act;

F . that the Articles are not hazardous substances or, if they are hazardous substances, are not misbranded hazardous substances or banned hazardous substances within the meaning of the Federal Hazardous Substances Act (including the former Federal Caustic Poison Act);

G . that all Articles furnished hereunder will be produced and sold in compliance with all applicable requirements of the Fair Labor Standards Act, as amended, including Sections 6, 7, and 12, and the regulations and orders issued under Section 14 thereof, and that it will certify such compliance on each invoice submitted in connection with this order;

H . that the Articles are not misbranded under the provisions of the Wool Products Labeling Act;

I . that it will comply with all applicable Equal Employment Opportunity requirements including those set forth in Section 202 of Executive Order 11246, as amended, which requirements are incorporated herein by reference;

J . that the Articles are not manufactured or sold in violation of the Occupational Safety and Health Act of 1970; and

K . that to the extent Seller is engaged in the marketing or handling of products, fabrics, or related material subject to the Flammable Fabrics Act, as amended, and regulations thereunder, Seller hereby guarantees to Buyer that with regard to all the products, fabrics, or related materials sold or to be sold to Buyer by

Seller, and for which flammability standards have been issued, amended, reasonable and representative tests as prescribed by the Federal Trade Commission have been performed that show that the products, fabrics, or related materials, at the time of their shipment or delivery by Seller, conform to such of the above-mentioned flammability standards as are applicable thereto. This guarantee shall also apply to any applicable codes of the National Fire Prevention Association (NFPA) and to any applicable state or local laws that are substantially identical to the Flammable Fabrics Act or that adopt the tests provided for in any applicable code of the NFPA.

Indemnity and Insurance. Seller shall defend, indemnify, and hold harmless Buyer, its employees, customers, and users of the Articles, from and against any claim, loss, damage, or expense arising out of the purchase and/or use of the Articles purchased hereunder and/or arising out of Seller's (or its subcontractor's) work or performance hereunder and shall procure and maintain liability insurance, with contractual liability coverage, with minimum limits of $250,000/$500,000/$100,000 or with such higher limits as Buyer shall reasonably request. Seller shall on or before delivery of the Articles purchased hereunder, furnish to Buyer a Certificate of Insurance evidencing the foregoing coverage and limits.

Seller shall defend, indemnify, and hold harmless Buyer from and against the assessment by any third party of any liquidated damages or proven actual damages arising out of the failure of Seller to timely deliver the Articles purchased hereunder.

Seller shall defend, indemnify, and hold harmless Buyer, its employees, customers, and users of the Articles from and against any claim, loss (including the cost of any Articles lost by libel, condemnation, or voluntary recall), damage, or expense arising out of any claim or finding by the United States of America, any state or local government, or any agency or instrumentality thereof that the Articles are not as herein guaranteed and warranted.

Setoff. Buyer may set off any amount due from Seller to any division or subsidiary of any participating buying group, whether or not under this order, against any amount due Seller hereunder.

Assignment. Seller shall not assign this order or any interest herein, including any performance or any amount that may be due or may become due hereunder, without Buyer's prior written consent.

Subcontracting. If any Articles are to be made to Buyer's design, all subcontracting by Seller with respect thereto shall be subject to Buyer's written approval.

Advertising. Seller shall not advertise or publish the fact that Buyer has placed this order without Buyer's prior written consent, except as may be necessary to comply with a proper request for information from an authorized representative of any governmental unit or agency.

Controlling Law. This order and the performance of the parties hereunder shall be controlled and governed by the law of the state shown in Buyer's address on the front side hereof.

Notice of Labor Disputes. Whenever an actual or potential labor dispute is delaying or threatens to delay the timely performance of this order, Seller shall immediately give notice thereof, including all relevant information with respect thereto, to Buyer. Seller shall insert the substance of this paragraph in any subcontract hereunder so that each such subcontract shall provide that in the event its timely performance is delayed or threatened by delay by any actual or potential labor dispute, the subcontractor shall immediately notify Seller of all relevant information with respect to such dispute.

Trademarks. Buyer warrants that all of the trademarks Buyer requests Seller to affix to the Articles purchased are those owned by Buyer and it is understood Seller shall not acquire or claim any rights, title, or interest therein, or use any of such trademarks on any Articles produced for itself or any one other than Buyer.

Risk of Loss. Risk of loss or damage to the Articles shall be on Seller until said Articles have been delivered to and accepted by Buyer, notwithstanding any other terms contained herein. All Articles will be received by Buyer subject to its right of inspection and rejection. Buyer shall be allowed a reasonable period of time to inspect the Articles and to notify Seller of any nonconformance with the terms and conditions of this order. Buyer may reject any Articles which do not conform to the terms and conditions of this order. Articles so rejected may be returned to Seller, or held by Buyer, at Seller's risk and expense.

Delivery of Goods. All shipments F.O.B.,

Kenosha Memorial Hospital, Kenosha, Wisconsin 53140. Shipment subject to cancellation if not delivered in time specified. Substitution not permitted without approval of materiel management department. Overshipments by Seller shall be subject to a $100 or 50 percent penalty, whichever is greater, which shall be deducted from that invoice. Goods not received by agreed on delivery date shall be subject to a penalty of $20 per line item, to be deducted from monthly statement. If the Seller is unable to deliver goods within the specified time period pursuant to a previously contracted price, the Seller shall be responsible for the difference between the contracted price and the price the Buyer is forced to pay when purchasing on the open market. This difference shall be charged directly to the Seller and deducted from the monthly statement.

Payment. Items received on or after the 25th of the month shall be considered as part of the following month's purchases. Invoice discounts will be taken until the 10th of the month following purchase. Total payment will be made upon installation and acceptance of equipment. No partial payment will be made, unless specifically so stated.

General. All warranties shall be construed as conditions as well as warranties. No waiver of a breach or of any provision of this order shall constitute a waiver of any other breach or provision. No modification, change in, departure from, or waiver of the provisions of this order shall be valid or binding unless approved by Buyer in writing. This order shall constitute the entire agreement between the parties.

Overcoming economic order quantity limitations

Peter C. Mike
Director
Materiel Management
L. W. Blake Memorial Hospital
Bradenton, Florida

Timothy W. Malburg
Graduate Student
Cornell University Graduate School of
    Business and Public Administration
Ithaca, New York

FOR YEARS scholars have acclaimed the advantages of using the economic order quantity (EOQ) to establish maximum order volume for supply inventories. Many materiel managers find the formula alone "mind boggling." In addition the following requirements may be necessary:

1. The unit price of each inventory item must be relatively stable.
2. The unit usage must be relatively stable.
3. Unlimited storage space must exist.

Although hospital purchasing managers appear to be holding their own on prices, requirements 2 and 3 are not usually met.

A method of EOQ calculation may be developed that is simple enough to be used by the inventory supervisor for all high dollar volume or "A" items on a periodic schedule. Restricting the application to "A" items only may reduce the impact on available storage space. The ability to recalculate rapidly may cushion the impact of fluctuations in usage.

CALCULATE COSTS

The development of a three-scale nomograph will provide the flexibility to overcome the limitations of the calculation and use of the EOQ. The following step-by-step approach may be used to develop a nomograph.

1. Develop an accurate identification of all costs involved in the economic order quantity formula.
2. Use the formula:

$$EOQ = \sqrt{\frac{2 \times \text{Annual Usage} \times \text{Purchase Order Cost}}{\text{Unit Cost} \times \text{Inventory Carrying Cost}}}.$$

Annual usage and unit costs

Annual usage and unit costs can be identified accurately by examining the inventory records that are usually kept by the inventory clerk. Where data have not been recorded on inventory sheets, the following steps may be taken:

1. Record data on usage for at least three months. A relatively simple format should be used. These data should be annualized. (The relative importance of defining usage, not just issues, should be kept in mind.)
2. Record the unit cost of item that is available directly from invoice copies either within the hospital or from the supplier.

Purchase order costs

Purchase order costs represent the total purchase order cost per line item. The first step is to determine personnel costs. A flow chart that identifies all personnel involved in processing purchase orders should be constructed. (Receiving and accounts payable personnel should not be overlooked.) The amount of time each employee spends processing a purchase order should be determined, then multiplied by his or her respective wage per hour. Together these personnel costs will give the total personnel cost per purchase order.

$$\sum_{i=1 \text{ (the index of summation)}}^{N \text{ (sample size)}} [(\text{employee's time/purchase order}) \times \text{employee's salary})]$$

The second step is to determine fringe benefits cost by multiplying the total personnel cost per purchase order by 12 percent. Fringe benefits of employees usually average around 12 percent of their salaries. In some geographical areas they may be as high as 20 percent of salaries.

The third step is to determine office supplies cost. The total volume of office supplies used can be located in the purchasing department's expense summary. The office supplies cost per purchase order can be determined by dividing the yearly office supplies expense by the total number of purchase orders per year. (Assuming that there is a constant demand, a purchase order log may be kept for three months to estimate the annual number of purchase orders processed.) Where a purchase order expense summary is not available these data may be obtained directly from purchase order copies, storeroom request copies, or vendor invoice copies. The last is the most difficult to trace to a particular cost center.

The fourth step is to determine utility and maintenance costs, using the hospital's cost worksheet. This worksheet usually

---

Formula to Determine Utility and Maintenance Costs

$$\text{Utility \& Maintenance Cost Per Purchase Order} = \text{Utility \& Maintenance Costs per Sq. Ft.} \times \frac{\text{Total Number of Sq. Ft. Utilized by Personnel Involved with Processing Purchase Orders}}{\text{Number of Purchase Orders Processed Yearly}}$$

---

contains a cost allocation method (i.e., step-down, double apportionment) that describes the costs of utility and maintenance on a square footage basis. The formula in boxed material above can be used.

The fifth step is to determine postage costs. Such costs are computed by dividing the annual number of purchase orders that require postage by the annual number of purchase orders processed, and multiplying that amount by $0.15. The materiel manager should ensure, however, that postal expenses have not already been included under office supplies costs.

The sixth step is to determine telephone costs. The purchasing department's telephone costs should have been itemized on its expense summary; in this case the same procedure as for office supplies cost should be followed. If this information is not available, a long distance log should be kept. The telephone company can be asked to supply a usage study to identify what calls were made and their respective toll costs. To determine telephone costs divide the purchasing department's total toll cost by the total numbers of purchasing orders processed during the toll usage study.

By adding the subtotals calculated in steps one through five, the total purchasing order costs can be derived. The purchase order cost per line item can be

obtained by dividing the total purchase costs by the average number of line items per purchase order.

Inventory carrying costs

Inventory carrying costs represent the total costs associated with holding inventories: (1) opportunity costs; (2) insurance and property tax costs; (3) storage costs; and (4) obsolescence, deterioration, and theft costs. These costs should be calculated as a percentage of the average inventory value. A breakdown of carrying costs is given in Table 1.

Opportunity costs

Hospitals that use leverage to purchase inventory items experience an opportunity cost of the interest rate on the borrowed funds. Hospitals that do not use leverage experience an opportunity cost of the insti-

Table 1. Breakdown of carrying costs

Carrying costs	Percent*
Interest Charges On Investment	7.25
Insurance Costs	1.00
Storage Costs	18.51
Obsolescence, Deterioration, Theft	1.00
Property Taxes	1.00
Total	28.76

*Percentages used are from L.W. Blake Memorial Hospital.

SCALE I	SCALE II	SCALE III
Monthly usage in units	Economic order quantity in units	Unit cost in dollars

Instructions

1. Locate the monthly usage of an inventory item on Scale I.

2. Locate the inventory item's unit purchase price on Scale III.

3. Using a straightedge connect the monthly usage on Scale I with unit cost on Scale III. The economic order quantity in units is read from the center scale at the point where it is crossed by the straightedge.

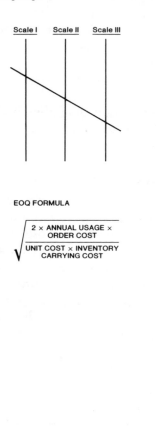

EOQ FORMULA

$$\sqrt{\frac{2 \times \text{ANNUAL USAGE} \times \text{ORDER COST}}{\text{UNIT COST} \times \text{INVENTORY CARRYING COST}}}$$

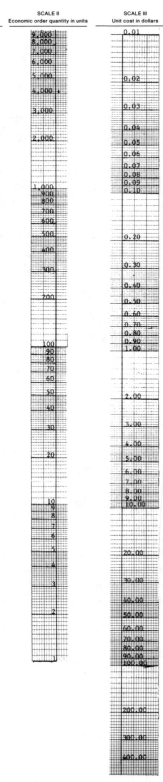

Figure 1. Using a nomograph. Note: Vertical positioning of the scales depends on the firm's actual order cost and inventory carrying cost. In this case the scales have been positioned based on: (1) order cost 24.97/order and/or 4.16/line item and (2) carrying cost of 28.67% of average inventory. Exact reduction ×3 (distance between scales—$1^{16}/_{32}''$ Cycle Distance—$3^{21}/_{64}''$).

tution's average rate of return on investments. If no investment projects are available the savings interest rate from local banks becomes the opportunity cost.

Insurance and property tax costs

Insurance and property tax costs are usually each conservatively estimated at one to three percent of average inventory value, depending on the dollar value of the inventory. If further accuracy is desired, the accounting department should be consulted for insurance policy details and property tax information.

Storage costs

Storage costs consist of utility, maintenance, and building depreciation. Utility and maintenance costs are calculated similarly to purchase order utility and maintenance costs, except the square feet area of inventory storage is used. Building depreciation is calculated by determining the annual building depreciation expense and multiplying this amount by the ratio of inventory storage area to total building area. Both costs are combined to ascertain storage costs.

Obsolescence, deterioration, and theft costs

Obsolescence, deterioration, and theft costs, combined, can usually be estimated at one to three percent, or can be deter-

mined by the percentage variance calculated at the last periodic inventory count.

The inventory carrying costs can be determined by adding the subtotals of the four kinds of inventory carrying costs.

CONSTRUCT A NOMOGRAPH

The three-scale nomograph consists of Scale I: Monthly Usage in Units; Scale II: EOQ in Units; and Scale III: Unit Costs in Dollars. These scales are composed of logarithmic cycles. A logarithmic cycle may begin with any number and end with a number ten times greater. By using the EOQ formula it was calculated that each scale will have an equal cycle length and be positioned equidistant from the other. Note, however, that Scale III, Unit Cost in Dollars, is inverted. The vertical positioning of Scales II and III can be determined by working a few numerical examples using the given EOQ formula. The proper calibrations for each cycle length can be obtained most easily with a slide rule or logarithmic graph paper. The use of nomographs is demonstrated in Figure 1.

The inventory supervisor may use the nomograph method of EOQ with relative ease. Restricting its application to high dollar volume items will reduce the effect on available storage space. The ability to recalculate rapidly will cushion the impact of fluctuations in usage.

SELECTED READINGS

Ammer, D. *Purchasing & Materials Management for Health Care Institutions* (Lexington, Mass.: D. C. Heath and Company 1976.)

Ammer, D. *Hospital Purchasing Management*. Editorial (June 1980).

Berman, H. and Weeks, L. *The Financial Management of Hospitals* (Ann Arbor: Health Administration Press 1979).

Knight, W. "Working Capital Management, Satisfying Versus Optimization." *Financial Management* (Spring 1972).

Levens, A. S. *Nomograph* (New York: John Wiley & Sons, Inc. 1959).

Miller, D. W. and Starr, M. *Inventory Control* (Englewood Cliffs, N.J.: Prentice Hall, Inc. 1962).

Purchasing for the small hospital

James C. Richardson
Director
Materiel Management
Centro Asturiano Hospital
Tampa, Florida

THOSE WHO ARE RESPONSIBLE for purchasing in small hospitals, regardless of their titles, often feel that they face unique problems. They all know that sending out requests for bids on small volume is frustrating, since vendors are usually interested in high-volume situations. Further, it is common knowledge that many small unaffiliated hospitals are regarded by some vendors as means to raise net profit figures. It seems that many small hospitals willingly pay full list price without question.

While money seems to be in tight supply everywhere, the private, not-for-profit, unendowed, unaffiliated hospitals suffer intensely. In many cases money for the upgrading and streamlining of services— and sometimes simply the cash flow for day-to-day operation—is not available on a continuing basis. Fulltime equivalents are perpetually in short supply. Purchasing agents have to "wear at least two hats." It is not uncommon for almost anyone to be the purchasing agent, and many small hospitals allow every department to do its own purchasing. This method creates havoc in every area of purchasing, from security to inventory control.

It is distressing that some consider these methods right and proper. The belief that the hospital can save money by building a warehouse so more can be purchased and inventory can be increased also exists. It is no surprise that cash flow problems result.

When all of these fallacies add up, the situation seems ominous. Anyone interested in rational purchasing systems might be expected to head for a large hospital. Purchasing for the small hospital appears to be hopeless.

ADVANTAGES OF SMALL HOSPITALS

With the proper attitude and philosophy, purchasing in the small institutional setting can be an exciting opportunity. A small hospital can develop a lean, hungry, and easy-to-maneuver posture quicker than the committee-strewn, glacier-like movements that typify the large hospital scene. While many will continue to argue that it is almost impossible for the smaller hospital to obtain consistently lower prices for goods and services, this idea should be permanently laid to rest. If as much time were spent exploring different methods of saving money as is spent lamenting that it cannot be done, more would be accomplished.

Small hospitals often have advantages over their larger counterparts. In many cases the small hospital is a source of public pride and support. Often services

and considerations are extended by local businesses and professionals who act as friends of the institution. This support can take many and varied forms, from special discounts and volunteer labor to donations for scholarships for nurses and other health care areas directly related to the hospital.

CENTRALIZED PURCHASING

Today many small hospitals are developing new purchasing programs based on the solid foundations of centralized purchasing, group purchasing, sound negotiations, and proper materiel management. In most small hospitals, department heads are, by necessity, technicians as well as supervisors. For this reason it becomes logical and beneficial for them to be free of the time-consuming function of purchasing to be able to devote those hours to departmental activities.

The program should begin by utilizing the expertise of those departments now doing purchasing to prepare specifications and guidelines for approved products,

The program should begin by utilizing the expertise of those departments now doing purchasing to prepare specifications and guidelines for approved products, services, and specific inventory amounts.

services, and specific inventory amounts. This is an important and basic step toward a smooth-running program. Only when this concept is understood and accepted will the value of centralized purchasing be realized.

The most important, and sometimes the most difficult, department to involve in centralized purchasing is pharmacy. Pharmacy traditionally has one of the highest inventories and budgets in the hospital. For this reason, especially in a small hospital, the pharmacist is a logical prospect for the purchasing/materiel management role. It must be emphasized that only the pharmacist with management skills and a desire to participate and cooperate in the various supply and purchasing activities is the proper candidate anywhere, but especially in a small hospital.

Gaining pharmacy's cooperation is essential because the whole program of centralized purchasing can be ineffectual if this large purchaser continues to have a high inventory and low turnover rate, and justifies this with, "We have always done it this way." The small hospital typically has a pharmacy inventory of $500 plus per bed and inventory turns of three to four times per year. By using a prime vendor concept with a local drug wholesaler, even a small hospital can negotiate excellent cost-plus pricing. Using this method, combined with favorable bids negotiated individually or through a buying group, and a comprehensive formulary (i.e., standardization of the use of certain drugs to lower inventory), pharmacy can lower its inventory to reflect at least ten turns a year while actually saving money on drug purchases. Under $200 per bed is easily obtainable for the typical hospital pharmacy.

The pharmacy in the 144-bed Centro Asturiano Hospital in Tampa, Florida includes an active outpatient section that fills true outpatient prescriptions, not generated by captive in-house clinics, allowing even closer inventory control. The pharmacy has been successful in lowering its inventory 46 percent in nine months using the centralized purchasing and prime vendor concepts. By using this process, inventory turns moved from 6.4 to just over 15. This was done at no increase in cost of purchase and with a low stock-out situation. It can be done! When it is done, less inventory means greater cash flow.

GROUP PURCHASING

Because of the proliferation of purchasing groups in most areas of the country, there is little excuse not to utilize their advantages. A small hospital should join a viable, progressive group and support it. Properly used, group purchasing can be the heart of a revitalized purchasing program. By using the expertise and buying power of the group, significantly lower prices can be obtained on goods and services, again releasing money for cash flow. Using available contracts can actually mean the difference between net profit and net loss at the end of the year.

Group purchasing can enhance the prime vendor concept. Obviously a vendor who will make price concessions for 90 percent of a small hospital's available business will probably make further discounts and services available to the group. The proper purchasing program will effect standardization. Properly negotiated contracts can lower costs in two ways—by improving acquisition prices and by allowing standardization to lower the number of items inventoried.

INVENTORY PRACTICES

Inventory dollars tied up in central stores can be released by faster turns. A small hospital practicing efficient purchasing can work on a two-week inventory, which would mean turning its inventory 26 times per year. Consignment, or the practice of having a manufacturer stock a commodity at the hospital but not charge for it until used, is a must for a hospital to eliminate the high dollar investment in such items as pacemakers and total hip replacements. The small hospital should immediately include consignment in its basic purchasing program.

PRINTING

Another area that typically demands immediate attention is printing. Usually a responsibility of central stores, printing is often a trouble area. Centro Asturiano Hospital's printing inventory was approaching $230 per occupied bed, but true to the then-accepted philosophy, this was considered proper because an extra discount (usually 5 percent) was obtained for quantity buying. In an ideal situation the print shop is added to the hospital, but if the money is not available, another method can be used successfully.

By using a prime vendor concept with a national firm and a local printer, Centro Asturiano was able to lower its printing inventory 74 percent in one year. It was actually able to operate all stores on little more than the same dollar volume printing had required 12 months previously. This is an example of how a small hospital can develop a lean and efficient attitude, and at the same time, release $20,000 for cash flow.

It is obvious that purchasing in a small hospital need not be the desolate scene that some would believe. New and enlightened methods can become the cornerstone of a revitalized purchasing program. When old fears and fallacies are discarded and new ideas are adopted, intelligent purchasing can become the first step toward a comprehensive and successful materiel management program.

Competitive bidding: an effective purchasing tool

William E. Pauley
Director, Shared Purchasing Programs
Multihospital Shared Services, Inc.
Marina del Rey, California

THE CURRENT climate of widespread concern over escalating health care costs has placed many new demands on the hospital administrator. The prudent administrator will take steps to ensure that the hospital's purchasing is done in a systematic manner that will help keep costs under control. Purchasing decisions should be able to withstand auditing and even public scrutiny. The best way to contain costs of supplies is to utilize competitive bidding. Effective use of this system can save the hospital thousands, and the health care industry millions of dollars each year.

THE PROBLEM

In order for a competitive bidding system to be instituted and successfully used to reduce costs, several typical problems must be overcome. The worst of these is the problem of decentralized purchasing. Many hospitals still permit 60 to 70 percent of total purchasing dollars to be expended by individual departments rather than a central purchasing department or the purchasing division of a materiel management department. The splitting of purchasing functions deprives the hospital of the advantage of its own purchasing volume, as well as savings that could be achieved through participation in group purchasing programs.

Another disadvantage of decentralized purchasing is that it allows suppliers to obtain undue influence over departmental purchases. Medical professionals cannot (and should not) give their full attention to product and cost evaluation, and thus are vulnerable to supplier pressure to deal with a sole source, making little or no comparison of products or prices. In addition, staff of the various departments are likely to develop personal preferences for products, backed up by an attitude that only their department is capable of purchasing the supplies needed. All these factors contribute to unnecessarily high costs.

THE SOLUTION

Centralized purchasing

The first step toward instituting a system of competitive bidding must be taken by the hospital's top management. One department, most likely materiel management, must be given control over purchasing. It must have full authority over the methods by which equipment, supplies, and services are purchased and it must be held accountable for performing this function in the most cost-effective manner.

Secondly, the materiel manager must develop a plan for systematic purchasing

and an appropriate organizational structure for implementing new practices. Top management support is again crucial if individual departments are to be weaned away from their enjoyment of autonomy and persuaded of the benefits of centralized purchasing.

Teamwork in developing product specifications

A team approach is imperative if competitive bidding is to be successful. The purchasing process must be organized so that input is obtained from the departments that will use the products and services. Just as a supplier maintains records of such information in order to provide efficient service, so materiel management should file for quick reference all the information received from the user departments.

The user department is best able to:

- furnish technical criteria and standards that materiel management can use as a basis for procurement specifications;
- evaluate supplies, equipment, and service performance so that specifications can be refined and better product choices made by materiel management; and
- review and select commonly used products for possible standardization,

---

Purchasing from a sole source, although more costly to the hospital, may at times be fully justified. However, it should be treated as an exception, not a routine practice.

---

so that the same brand will be used for the same or similar functions.

Frequently, a user will express a preference for the product of a particular supplier. Materiel management will have to determine whether this is merely a personal preference left over from the days of autonomous departmental purchasing, or whether it reflects a real difference in the performance capability of different products. The user should be asked to substantiate the preference by identifying specific problems with other brands. Purchasing from a sole source, although more costly to the hospital, may at times be fully justified. However, it should be treated as an exception, not a routine practice.

Materiel management should prepare a checklist, such as the one shown in Figure 1, to be used in preparing the specifications for a formal request for bids. If any item applicable to the product in question is not addressed, the result will be added cost for the hospital. Oversights that must be corrected later always involve additional expense.

Securing bids or quotations

The hospital should maintain a list of acceptable sources for bidding, quotations, and negotiating purposes by utilizing either a bidder's list application or vendor information form on which data pertaining to the vendor are recorded and kept current. (See Appendix.) Such lists should be kept current by adding new sources and deleting sources that have not been active participants in the hospital's buying process or have not participated in the hospital's cost-reduction program.

Spec req (verify & include prior to purchase)
- ☐ Accessories (itemize)
- ☐ Capacity
- ☐ Color
- ☐ Electrical
- ☐ Finish
- ☐ Flammability
- ☐ Heating
- ☐ Inspection & acceptance (by whom)
- ☐ Installation (by whom)
- ☐ Options
- ☐ Plumbing
- ☐ Refrigeration
- ☐ Repair source
- ☐ Safety (OSHA, etc.)
- ☐ Service manuals, schematics, shop drawings
- ☐ Size
- ☐ Space
- ☐ Spare parts inventory (itemize)
- ☐ Special requirements (itemize)
- ☐ Supplies required (initially and ongoing— itemize)
- ☐ Technical data (wiring diagrams schematics, shop drawings, etc.)
- ☐ Training (in-service, factory, etc.)
- ☐ Upholstery
- ☐ Warranty
- ☐ Weight

Figure 1. Specification checklist.

Bids or quotations should be requested from a firm only with the intent of doing business. Submitting bids and quotations is an expense, and it is unethical to ask a vendor to prepare them when no contract or order will be made regardless of the price quoted. Price should be the only unknown factor at the time bids or quotations are requested. Materiel management should have already investigated the vendor's quality, delivery, and service capabilities. However, when buying an item from a new vendor with whom there has been no prior experience, investigation can wait until a favorable bid or quotation has been submitted.

One of the most frequent complaints

How many sources should be invited to bid or quote? The answer depends on the value of the purchase and how much knowledge materiel management has of the marketing system of the items to be purchased.

registered by sellers is that bids and requests for quotations do not clearly communicate product specifications, terms, conditions, and delivery to be met. Filling out this information requires an exchange of correspondence or telephone calls, and makes the vendor wonder how the hospital can make a fair evaluation to determine contract award or order placement. Another complaint is that often the closing date does not allow the vendor time for proper preparation and leads to a hastily produced bid. If such poor planning is practiced by the hospital's materiel management, the use of competitive bidding adds to the cost an unnecessary administrative expense, and results in a poor business image.

How many sources should be invited to bid or quote? The answer depends on the value of the purchase and how much knowledge materiel management has of the marketing system of the items to be purchased. The main concern here is the selection of a source that will remove any doubts concerning price, quality, quantity, or delivery. The number can vary from 2 sources to 20 or more. Marketing knowledge obtained from such coverage should be maintained in an approved-vendor file, so as to have it available for future use.

A standard form, such as that shown in Figure 2, should be used for bid requests.

Additional pages can be attached if bids are sought for more items. Also, it is most efficient to use a standard form to keep a concise record of bids received. (See Figure 3). Again, additional pages can be added as needed. These records can be produced manually as in Figures 2 and 3, or by computer as in Figure 4. Preprinted bid sheets, computer or manual, for such items as produce, fresh meat, and frozen food can be used to expedite the buying of items where the price fluctuates frequently.

Standard items needed for day-to-day operations such as stationery, laundry supplies, medical and surgical supplies, electrical and plumbing supplies, etc., which are normally sold on the basis of catalog prices, can be obtained by placing annual contracts. In most cases a trade discount can be obtained by requesting bids once a year and including in the contract a price escalation clause that allows prices to change in an auditable manner. Purchase orders can then be placed during the contract period as needs arise. Bakery and dairy products can best be obtained by annual bidding. The main concern here is economical acquisition at the least overhead expense possible.

Buying routine items by such methods will provide time for materiel management personnel to function more effectively in the acquisition of capital items and in other areas. With too much time spent in routine purchases, the large expenditures could cost the hospital more because materiel management skills could not be adequately utilized in this area.

Suppliers should be encouraged to offer substitutes and additional suggestions to items specified in the bid or request for

THIS REQUEST ISSUED BY:

MULTIHOSPITAL SHARED SERVICES, INC.
4676 ADMIRALTY WAY, SUITE 426
MARINA DEL REY, CALIFORNIA 90291
TELEPHONE (213) 823-0947

mssi REQUEST FOR QUOTATION

DATE ISSUED	QUOTATION NO.	PAGE
		OF

THIS IS AN INQUIRY, NOT AN ORDER

REPLY DUE BY (Closing Date)	←

QUOTATION REQUESTED BY (NAME AND TITLE)	ADDRESS REPLY TO:
SIGNATURE	

Request quotation for furnishing the following equipment, supplies and/or services for delivery of equipment or supplies at the F.O.B. point indicated or performance of service at the job site location as indicated herein.

DELIVERY: Equipment, supplies or services desired no later than _____ . Indicate your best possible delivery or performance time_____.

SUBMISSION OF QUOTATION (BID): One completed copy must be returned by above closing date _____ . Order(s) will be placed within _____ days from opening date. Name of firm receiving order(s) will be furnished upon request.

SPECIFICATIONS: Equipment, supplies, or services per specifications set forth herein or as attached.

TERMS AND CONDITIONS: As set forth herein or as attached. A copy or Vendor's Warranty to be supplied with quotation

ITEM NO.	QUANTITY	UNIT	DESCRIPTION	QUOTED UNIT PRICE	QUOTED TOTAL AMOUNT
			Your suggestions for lower costs are solicited.		

The undersigned hereby quotes prices for furnishing any or all of the items opposite which prices are shown, delivered at the point specified or performance of service at the job site location and within the time indicated. Price will remain firm for _____ days. Discount will be allowed as follows: _____ percent 10 days; _____ percent 20 days; _____ percent 30 days. Other: _____
_____ ☐ Regular Dealer   ☐ Manufacturer   ☐ Repair Facility   ☐ Other (specify) _____

My Quote No._____   Date _____   F.O.B. _____

Shipping Point_____   Service Performance Location_____
(If more than one destination point indicate opposite each item on which an offer is made)

Name of Bidder_____   Name and Title of Person Authorized To Sign Bids (Offers)_____

Address_____   Signature_____

Wats Line (Toll Free) No._____   Title _____

Phone No. _____

Figure 2. Sample request for quotation. Source: Multihospital Shared Services, Inc. Reprinted with permission.

MULTIHOSPITAL SHARED SERVICES, INC.
4676 ADMIRALTY WAY, SUITE 426
MARINA DEL REY, CALIFORNIA 90291

FACILITY:_____

PURCHASE ORDER/CONTRACT NUMBER	PURCHASE AUTHORITY (Hospital P.O., etc.)	**QUOTATION RECORD AND WORK SHEET**		SHEET NUMBER	NR OF SHEETS

(Form: Quotation Record and Work Sheet, with fields including DATE OF ORDER, DATE(S) DELIVERY, SHIP TO, BIDDER NUMBER 1, BIDDER NUMBER 2; DELIVERY F.O.B. ☐ DESTINATION ☐ OTHER (SPECIFY); DISCOUNT TERMS, TYPE OF ORDER ☐ PURCHASE DELIVERY ORDER ☐ MSSI NATIONAL AGREEMENT ☐ ORAL (Confirming Order) ☐ WRITTEN; TO (CONTRACTOR AND ADDRESS); BIDDER NUMBER 3, BIDDER NUMBER 4; DATE OF QUOTE; ACCOUNT NUMBER CHARGEABLE; AWARDED TO BIDDER NUMBER:)

ITEM NBR	SUPPLIES OR SERVICES	QUANTITY	UNIT	BIDDER NUMBER 1	BIDDER NUMBER 2	BIDDER NUMBER 3	BIDDER NUMBER 4

BUYER	CHECKERS INIT.	TYPIST'S INIT	DELIVERY DATE				
			DISCOUNT				
☐ CONFIRMATION ORDER	☐ DELIVERY ORDER NATIONAL AGREEMENT		F.O.B. DESTINATION				
REMARKS			F.O.B. OTHER - SPECIFY				
			TYPE OF QUOTE				
BUYER			PERSON CONTACTED				
SIGNATURE AUTHORIZATION			QUOTE DATE				

REASON FOR P.O./CONTRACT AWARD:	☐ LOWEST PRICE AT SAME QUALITY	☐ BEST DELY SCHEDULE (ONLY WHEN DELY IS OF PRIME IMPORTANCE)	☐ OTHER (EXPLAIN):

Figure 3. Quotation record. Source: Multihospital Shared Services, Inc. Reprinted with permission.

quotation. To make this possible, it is necessary to furnish the function or the performance required along with the item's specifications. Supplying performance information can also encourage suppliers to utilize their skills in a cost-reduction program.

COMPETITIVE BIDDING VERSUS NEGOTIATION

The hospital should publish a policy statement that indicates its concern about costs by stating that it will use a formal system of competitive bidding whenever feasible, and that procurement by negotiation is an exception requiring prior authorization. Negotiation with a single vendor is much less likely than competitive bidding to result in the lowest price for an item. To say that a price from only one vendor is fair and reasonable requires knowledge of the supplier's marketing strategy, operations, and other phases of business—expertise that is rarely available to a hospital.

However, there are some cases, often involving purchases of highly technical equipment, in which negotiation must be used because competitive bidding is not

```
                MULTIHOSPITAL SHARED SERVICES, INC.

                   DRUG BID LIST - FOR MAY 1, 1981                      3 7
--------------------------------------------------------------------------------
   PRODUCT DESCRIPTION AND          ESTIMATED   BRAND NAME* OR      BID PRICE PER UNIT
      SPECIFICATIONS                QUANTITY      ALTERNATE         DIRECT        DEPOT
--------------------------------------------------------------------------------
2405193-------------------------------------------------------------------------
   XYLOCAINE INJECTION    5 ML                      •
             1 %           AMP        9,900.                          •            •
2405173-------------------------------------------------------------------------
   XYLOCAINE INJECTION   20 ML                      •
             1 %           V          3,960.                          •            •
2405273-------------------------------------------------------------------------

             2 %           V          1,200.        •                •            •
2405153-------------------------------------------------------------------------
   XYLOCAINE INJECTION   30 ML MDV                  •
             1 %           B          1,440.                          •            •
2405143-------------------------------------------------------------------------
   XYLOCAINE INJECTION   50 ML MDV                  •
             1 %           B          2,080.                          •            •
2405243-------------------------------------------------------------------------

             2 %           B          1,024.        •                •            •
2405147-------------------------------------------------------------------------
   XYLOCAINE JELLY - 30 ML                          •
             2 %           B          2,940.                          •            •
2410193-------------------------------------------------------------------------
   XYLOCAINE W/EPINEPHRINE INJECTION   20 ML.
             1 %           AMP        3,615.                          •            •
2410173-------------------------------------------------------------------------
   XYLOCAINE W/EPINEPHRINE INJECTION   30 ML.
             1 %           V          1,200.                          •            •
--------------------------------------------------------------------------------
```

```
--------------------------------------------------------------------------------
  *PLEASE IDENTIFY THE BRAND NAME YOU BID,
     IF APPLICABLE
                                         --------------------------------------
  BID ON ANY PACKAGE SIZE IN YOUR CATALOG,           FIRM
     BUT PLEASE INDICATE THE SIZE YOU BID.

  SIGNATURE CONSTITUTES ACCEPTANCE OF ALL  ------------------------------------
     RULES AND REGULATIONS CONTAINED IN THIS BID.    SIGNATURE
```

Figure 4. Computer-produced bid request sheet. Source: Multihospital Shared Services, Inc. Reprinted with permission.

practical, such as:

- when sources are limited; or
- when prices are fixed because of patents, fair trade, customs of the trade, or collusion.

When negotiation is necessary, it should be carried out by a special team including the materiel manager and the technical department manager. The latter should not handle the negotiations alone, as occurs in many hospitals, because more than just technical aspects must be considered if a reasonable price is to be obtained.

If the competitive bidding system is intelligently used, and if the bids and quotes are analyzed prior to issuing a purchase order or entering into a contract, then the hospital can be assured of receiving reasonable prices. This is true because the system, used properly, evaluates pricing factors bearing on the purchase being made. These factors include vendor efficiency, vendor willingness to price at a given profit level, and competitive conditions in general.

Sample vendor information form
Multihospital Shared Services, Inc.

(Hospital Heading)

Buying
Class

Vendor code no. _____

     Active

     Inactive

     Date _____ (explain)

VENDOR INFORMATION
(Bid list/source data)

Data of firms desiring to do business with _____

(TYPE OR PRINT CLEARLY)   Date _____

Company Name _____

Street Address _____

City, State, Zip Code _____

Telephone No. _____

WATS Line _____

Telex Twx No. _____

Purchase order/contract address if different than above _____

Payment/remittance address if different _____

Commodities/service handled _____

Catalog on file _____ . How long in business _____

References as to performance: Names of at least two hospitals other than _____
_____ preferred.

Category:

        ☐ Manufacturer   ☐ Stocking Dealer
        ☐ Nonstocking Dealer   ☐ Mfr. Representative
        ☐ Service Establishment ☐ Other Specify

Location of nearest full line stocking warehouse _____

Terms _____

Normal lead time to process and ship orders or perform service (days) _____

Insurance Coverage: (certificate required to be on file, kept current if vendors' personnel would ever work on or be on the premises or property of) _____

_____

_____

Other comments/remarks _____

Product liability insurance coverage—certificate required to be on file and kept current as long as vendor provides products to _____

PERSONS TO CONTACT

1. Sales Representative (name) _____
   Address _____
   Telephone No. _____

2. Authorized to quote prices _____
   Sign bids and contracts _____

3. Order placement _____

4. Errors in invoices _____

5. Delinquent orders/contracts _____

6. Damages and shortages in shipment _____

7. Quality _____

8. Claims _____

9. Vendor performance/improvement _____

10. Customer service _____

FREIGHT CHARGES

☐ F.O.B. Hospitals _____ _____ _____

☐ F.O.B. Shipping point _____

☐ Freight allowed on _____ lbs or more

☐ Other as specified

_____

_____

_____

Vendor performance rating _____

Annual $ Volume _____ from (date) _____ to (date) _____

Remarks: (response time/attention to matters, timely submission of B bids, etc.) _____

_____

Date vendor approved as a source: _____

If not approved or removed explain: _____

_____

_____

Corporate Director
Materiel Management

Development of a prudent purchasing program

Jerry P. Widman, J.D.
Manager
Ernst and Whinney
Cleveland, Ohio

TODAY'S ENVIRONMENT

THE SINGLE most important problem confronting all health care providers today is the rising cost of their daily operations.

Government figures indicate that the average person's health care bill has grown two and one-half times faster than average wage levels over the past 20 years. Major corporations are paying well over $1,500 per employee for hospital and medical care. In spite of the Voluntary Effort, the inflationary spiral within the health care segment of the economy continues to be a problem. Many explanations—such as the dramatic technological achievements in and the extraordinary quality of health care today—are offered for these rising costs.

As a result of improved employee benefits, many of the nation's families have unlimited access to the health care delivery system. Nonetheless, health care is costly. Purchasers of hospital services—including the federal government—are looking hard at these spiraling costs. Pressures on health care institutions for cost containment are intense and will become more intense. Most administrators today recall the fact that provisions of the economic stabilization program continued to apply to hospitals after similar controls were relaxed for the major portion of the economy in January 1973.

Hospital purchases are currently increasing at a rate greater than the overall cost of living. Two basic factors contribute to this increase: First, as with any business in today's economy, unit prices for hospital supplies are increasing. There is some evidence to support the fact that these increases are greater than other commodities within our economy. The other factor contributing to the rapid increase in the cost of hospital purchases is the increased *use* of supplies by hospitals.

Third party payers are becoming increasingly concerned with the costs of supplies, equipment and services. The more blatantly out-of-line the costs involved, as compared to the amount paid for similar goods and services, the more likely it is that the third party payer will challenge those costs. The basis of that challenge is the prudent buyer concept.

The prudent buyer concept has been in existence for several years. When it was first introduced it caused considerable excitement and anxiety within hospitals because of its potential threat to reimbursement. After a time, the excitement and anxiety diminished and very little was said or written about the prudent buyer concept. Recently, this "sleeping giant" has begun to stir again. More and more

intermediaries are requesting documentation of purchasing decisions and concentrating on auditing the costs of supplies, equipment and services.

It is important to note that for every 10 percent increase in wages and fringe benefits, the nonwage cost increases by 15 percent. Supplies and equipment are an important part of nonwage costs. In looking at practices relating to supplies and equipment, there are many hospitals with decentralized purchasing, but there are few hospitals with a genuinely centralized purchasing function. Despite the fact that the purchasing department itself usually accounts for less than one percent of the typical hospital's expenses, it is responsible for as much as 20 percent of the total cost. The purchasing department normally plays a limited role in the purchase of drugs and frequently has no role in dietary (food) supplies. Although many departments perform their own purchasing and inventory functions, purchasing is an insignificant portion of the overall activities of that particular department.

COST-CONTAINMENT LEGISLATION

On March 6, 1979 the Secretary of HEW sent the Congress a draft of legislation entitled the "Hospital Cost Containment Act of 1979." This bill was designed—

> ...to establish voluntary limits on the annual increases and total hospital expenses and to provide mandatory limits in the annual increases in hospital inpatient revenues to the extent that the voluntary limits are not effective.

The bill was introduced in the Senate by

Senator Gaylord Nelson (D-Wis.)[1] and in the House of Representatives by Representatives Charles Rangel (D-N.Y.) and Henry Waxman (D-Cal.).[2] The proposed legislation is the most recent in a series of congressional actions aimed at controlling the health care industry in this country. The bill has significant implications for health care providers with respect to Medicare, Medicaid and Blue Cross. If it is enacted, the basic principles, if not the mechanics, will certainly be included in any future expansion of the federal role in health care.

MEDICARE:
A THIRD PARTY PAYER

Medicare is the governmental program enacted in 1965 as Title XVIII of the Social Security Act.[3] It is designed to provide certain health care services required by the nation's elderly and disabled. Because of the large number of

> *Medicare is designed to provide the most penetrating short-term health care required by the nation's elderly and disabled.*

such beneficiaries and the scope of the program, Medicare affects many health care providers (e.g., hospitals, nursing homes, etc.).

Many analogies have been drawn between the development of Medicare reimbursement regulations and the development of the Internal Revenue Code. For example, both require the application of

generally accepted accounting principles in the determination of allowable (deductible) costs and expenses; both then proceed to list a number of exceptions. In addition, both have some logical inconsistencies due to the political and legislative process with its amendments, overlays and adjustments.

Unlike recent tax legislation, however, the Medicare legislation is rarely specific in administrative matters. Instead, Congress delegated an unusually broad scope of administrative authority to the Secretary of HEW for the purpose of furthering the implicit and explicit intent of the legislation. The powers of the secretary under the proposed cost-containment legislation indicate that this trend is likely to continue. Regulations promulgated by the secretary have the force of law as long as they are consistent with legislative purpose. The law as amended and its legislative history are therefore the foundation upon which the regulations and other interpretive pronouncements are based.

Interpretations of legislative intent— especially in politically sensitive areas involving public funds—generally lead to disagreements. Medicare reimbursement is no exception. Political pressures occasionally result in attempts to implement change through regulation or administrative channels at the limit or beyond the scope of delegated authority. In an effort to avoid the lengthy legislative process, Medicare reimbursement determinations are becoming case-based (case-by-case rather than amending the law for different situations).

In order to understand and appreciate the prudent buyer concept, one must be familiar with certain cost reimbursement aspects and the congressional intent behind cost reimbursement. A careful reading of the Senate Finance Committee reports pertaining to this legislation reveals the intent of Congress at the time the law was enacted.

Some of the key elements of congressional intent which affect cost reimbursement are:

1. paying all costs for program beneficiaries and none for other beneficiaries;

2. paying actual cost, without regard to how these costs may vary from one institution to another, unless the costs (in the aggregate) are substantially in excess of those costs incurred by similarly situated institutions in the same general geographic area;

3. paying costs when incurred;

4. following existing patterns of third-party reimbursement (both as to allowable cost and method of reimbursement);

5. providing a local alternative to centralized governmental bureaucracy through the use of "intermediaries;" and

6. relying upon the HEW secretary to issue all regulations appropriate to the implementation of the congressional mandate.

These are the elements of legislative intent which form the basis of today's reimbursement of costs to providers of health care under the Medicare program. Over the years other third party payers have seen fit to accept them.

FINANCIAL IMPLICATIONS FOR SUPPLY COSTS

Health care providers are reimbursed by five general classes of payer which include (1) Medicare, (2) Medicaid, (3) Blue Cross, (4) private insurance and (5) self-paying patients. Therefore cost savings which accrue directly to a provider from a specific cost reduction vary, depending on the reimbursement methods.

Under the current reimbursement plan, the true benefit of any cost savings is a function of the percent of the total reimbursement coming from *each* of the five payer classes. For example, Medicare and Medicaid generally reimburse based on cost with some ceilings. Therefore, reductions in the supply costs generally tend to reduce total reimbursement from Medicare and Medicaid. This saves money for the government and lowers the overall cost of health care. Because the provider is paid for its costs, the financial impact is not felt by the provider itself and the common attitude is: "Why bother?" Here are some reasons.

- Some hospitals experience costs which exceed Medicare inpatient routine cost limitations. Thus a hospital in this situation will lose reimbursement dollars. The loss of reimbursement dollars eventually creates cash-flow problems for the hospital that can lead to bankruptcy.

- Some hospitals' costs are in excess of charges and Medicare and Medicaid reimbursement may be based on charges. Because these excess costs are not reimbursed the provider never recovers its total costs.

- Private insurance companies and self-pay patients pay hospitals at predetermined charge levels. To the extent that costs exceed these predetermined levels, the provider does not "cover" costs.
- Some portion of the hospital's cost may be incurred in areas which are outside of any reimbursement consideration.

In many of the above situations, dollars saved by cost reductions flow directly to the bottom levels of the institution and may mean the difference between profit and loss.

The bases for Blue Cross reimbursement plans vary from plan to plan. Nationwide, there are about 65 Blue Cross plans. Of these, approximately one-half are cost-based reimbursement plans, one-third are charge-payment plans and the remainder fall in the prospective reimbursement category. With a passage of time and with ever-increasing costs, it is reasonable to assume that the percentage of plans relying solely on cost-based reimbursement will decrease. The effect will be that it behooves the provider to pay particular attention to its purchasing program and the cost effectiveness of that program.

THE REIMBURSEMENT PROCESS: A SHIFT IN EMPHASIS

During the past three decades, the health care industry has spent considerable sums of money on construction and renovation programs aimed at additional services and improved facilities. These expansion and rebuilding programs were followed by higher levels of operating costs. As the nation's hospital costs rose, the concept of "full" reimbursement for costs shifted toward the concept of *allowable* versus *nonallowable* costs. New reimbursement programs were tested and some were implemented—all with an emphasis on reducing the rate of increase of dollars paid to the provider of health care services. Thus it is more difficult today to maintain financial viability. Prospective reimbursement programs, cost ceilings, rate review commissions, etc., are all aimed at instilling within the hospital itself the concept of better management of its resources—including supplies and equipment. There is increased interest in improving cost effectiveness which is ultimately aimed at reducing cost or at least avoiding cost increases.

One objective of the health care reimbursement process is the determination of the allowable direct operating cost of each department within the particular health care institution. To accomplish this objective, the principles of reimbursement are applied to the expense data, and appropriate reclassifications and adjustments are made. The output of this initial phase is the "allowable" direct cost of operating each department. This cost is then subjected to cost finding and cost apportionment; and finally the net settlement is determined. To be considered "allowable," a provider's incurred cost must be reasonable and related to patient care.

Under the Medicare regulations, providers are generally reimbursed for the reasonable cost of services provided to Medicare beneficiaries. But what is "reasonable cost"? The answer lies in an examination of the regulations.

The following definition is an excerpt from the Social Security Act.

The reasonable cost of any services shall be the cost actually incurred excluding therefrom any part of incurred cost found to be unnecessary in the efficient delivery of needed health services, and shall be determined in accordance with regulations establishing the method or methods to be used, and the items to be included, in determining such costs for various types or classes of institutions . . . .[4]

This definition is expanded in the Medicare regulations.

All payments to providers of services must be based on the reasonable cost of services covered under Title XVIII of the Act and

---

Under the Medicare regulations, providers are generally reimbursed for the reasonable cost of services provided to Medicare beneficiaries. But what is "reasonable cost"?

---

related to the care of beneficiaries. Reasonable cost includes all necessary and proper costs incurred in rendering the services, subject to principles relating to specific items of revenue and cost . . . .[5]

The common term *necessary and proper* is used to describe what the concept of reasonable cost covers. This same section begins to indicate how the reasonable cost principle is to be applied:

However, where the provider's operating cost includes amounts not related to patient care, specifically not reimbursable under the program, or flowing from the provision of luxury items or services (that is, those items or services substantially in excess of

or more expensive than those generally considered necessary for the provision of needed health services), such amounts will not be allowable.[6]

THE PRUDENT BUYER PRINCIPLE

By now it should be clear that the key to which costs the provider will be reimbursed relates to the reasonable cost principle. The objective of most third party payers is to bear the costs (direct and indirect) of health care related to individuals covered by a particular health care program. The typical third party payer program will not pay the costs of health care attributable to individuals not covered by the program. Increased attention is being given to the costs attributable to individuals covered by a program such as Medicare.

The Health Care Financing Administration's *Medicare Provider Reimbursement Manual* contains a section which has gained increased application as the phrase *cost containment* becomes a part of the health care vocabulary. That section states:

Implicit in the intention that the actual costs be paid to the extent they are reasonable is the expectation that the provider seeks to minimize its costs and that its actual costs do not exceed what a prudent and cost-conscious buyer pays for a given item or service. If costs are determined to exceed the level that such buyers incur, in the absence of clear evidence that the higher costs were unavoidable, the excess costs are not reimbursable under the program.[7]

This section is the genesis of what is now

known as the "Prudent Buyer Principle." Simply stated, it means that the provider must act as a prudent and cost-conscious buyer. It must attempt to minimize costs in the purchase of supplies, equipment and services. To the extent that it fails to meet the duty of a prudent purchaser, it can expect to have a portion of its costs disallowed. The standard by which the hospital is to be judged is that of a prudent and cost-conscious buyer. In short, excess and unreasonable costs will be disallowed.

The application goes far beyond the purchase price of supplies, equipment and other materials. The prudent buyer concept has been the rationale used in numerous arguments concerning the allowability of costs. It is incorporated into many appeal arguments heard before the Provider Reimbursement Review Board regarding the allowability of various costs and is often cited in the rationale underlining that board's decision. As such, the authority given to the concept is greater than what is usually accorded interpretations of regulations.

Applications of the Prudent Buyer Concept

The prudent buyer concept has been applied to all of a particular cost or to a portion of that cost. Examples of application of this concept are found in virtually every facet of allowable costs. A few illustrations involve the allowability of the—

1. cost of underutilized in-house data processing equipment when the same services could have been purchased at half the cost from a service bureau

(allowability would depend on the hospital's individual situation);

2. cost of a physician contract which provides that the physician act in some administrative capacity (generally the contract must indicate the specific administrative duties in order for the provider to recoup those costs above the normal compensation); and

3. imputed savings from quantity and cash discounts which were readily available to the hospital but were not taken. This generally results in an offset of these unrealized savings unless the hospital can demonstrate extenuating circumstances).

The prudent and cost-conscious buyer not only refuses to pay more than the "going price" for an item, but also minimizes costs. The buyer as an institutional organization frequently purchases in large quantities. Often that buyer can obtain discounts due to the volume of its purchases. In addition, large purchases of single items usually lead to increased leverage in bargaining with individual suppliers for other items. Under the Medicare program, providers of health care services are expected to take advantage of such opportunities or to justify the reasons for any excess costs attributable to the failure to act as a prudent and cost-conscious buyer.

The obvious question becomes: how can such a nebulous concept ever be put into practice? The *Provider Reimbursement Manual* states:

Application of Prudent Buyer Principle—
Intermediaries may employ various means for detecting and investigating situations in

which costs seem excessive. Included may be such techniques as comparing the prices paid by providers to the prices paid for similar items or services by comparable purchasers, spot checking and inquiring providers about indirect, as well as direct, discounts. In addition, where a group of institutions has a joint purchasing arrangement which seems to result in participating members getting lower prices because of the advantage gained from bulk purchasing, any potentially eligible providers in the area which do not participate in the group may be called upon to justify any higher prices paid. Also when most of the costs of a service are reimbursed by Medicare (for a home health agency which treats only Medicare beneficiaries, for example), the cost should be examined with particular care. In those instances where an intermediary notes that a provider pays more than the going price for a supply or service in the absence of a clear justification for the premium, the intermediary will exclude excess cost in determining allowable costs under Medicare.[8]

A technique used by some intermediaries is to prove that a provider is not a prudent buyer of goods and services by a comparison approach. If area hospitals are of similar size and prove similar services receive discounts, then it is reasonable to expect the hospital in question should also receive such discounts. In reaching a final settlement figure, the third-party auditor may adjust the amount due to the hospital, to the extent that the hospital failed to take such discounts.

Another technique involves comparison of prices paid by Hospital "A" with those available through the local group purchasing organization. Once the comparison tests have been made, the third party payer discusses these price comparisons with the purchasing agent of Hospital "A." Strangely enough, large variances require justification for the variance. If the provider is unable or unwilling to show evidence of a plan or intent to obtain prices more in keeping with the group purchasing price, the third party payer is likely to consider an adjustment in the amount paid to Hospital "A."

There is a degree of uncertainty within the health care community as to what extent the government will implement the prudent buyer concept. However, experience with the Medicare program indicates that its provisions are likely to be

---

There is a degree of uncertainty within the health care community as to what extent the government will implement the prudent buyer concept.

---

expanded in the interest of cost containment. The fact is that hospital purchasing activities are not immune from numerous government controls. One theory being speculated about is that if a hospital does not buy from the lowest-priced vendor and is unable to adequately justify its choice, the third party may not pay any costs in excess of the lowest price. It is in the best interest of the institution to be able to demonstrate that it follows a prudent buyer program in the purchase of supplies, equipment and services.

The Prudent Buyer Program

While the prudent and cost-conscious buyer is not clearly defined, a sound purchasing program indicating conduct in keeping with a prudent buyer program should be in place. And while every provider need not demonstrate full implementation, any hospital addressing the prudent buyer problem should consider:

- written policies and procedures which govern the management of supplies, equipment and outside services;
- periodic product evaluation and standardization of commonly used items;
- use of competitive bidding;
- control over pilferage and obsolescence;
- evaluation of vendor performance with respect to price, quality and service;
- proper internal control practices and procedures relating to purchase, receipt and distribution of items as well as the payment of vendors;
- purchase orders with clear and explicit language covering the terms and conditions;
- participation in group purchasing activities wherever appropriate;
- documentation of current vendor quotations, price history records and supportive documents which authorize the buying action;
- investigation, approval and selection of sources of supply with due consideration to price, quality, availability and delivery;
- purchasing functions which are clearly assigned to specific individuals; and

- requisitioning process predicated on an appropriate level of supervision and approval.

Because the application of the prudent buyer concept is relatively new to the purchasing field, there appears to be no magic list or "generally accepted" methodology to determine whether or not an institution is in compliance with that concept. However, a hospital can invest in a review to identify the strengths and limiting factors of its purchasing activities with respect to the prudent buyer principle. Whether such a review is conducted internally (as a self-review) or by an outside consultant is a matter of choice.

Regardless of who conducts a review or evaluation of purchasing practices, certain techniques or approaches will most likely be followed. These include:

- interviewing purchasing employees and key members of user departments;
- examining the contents and design of key documents and records;
- evaluating the functional goals, policies and procedures of materiel management; and
- conducting random samples of selected records and documents.

Specific review steps for purchase transactions might include:

1. Determining the filing practices for all basic purchasing documents (e.g., requisitions, quotations, purchase orders, purchase order revisions, purchase history records).
2. Conducting a purchase order review by obtaining a representative sample of purchase orders over the past

12-month period. The representative sample should be a cross-section by buyer, by commodity category, by dollar value, by user department, etc.

3. Pulling all documents related to each purchase and preparing a worksheet to evaluate each of the purchase orders under consideration.

The objective of reviewing purchase transactions is to determine whether sound purchasing practices are being followed: Are the actions those of a prudent and cost-conscious buyer?

With the increasing inflationary pressures on today's health care industry, no institution can long afford to ignore the prudent buyer concept. Providers at the present time have a significant investment in inventory, and the cost of supplies, equipment and services is considered a major expense. On a comparative basis, supply costs are increasing at a rapid pace. In fact published statistics indicate that nonlabor costs are rising at a faster rate than labor costs. Part of this increase can be attributed to the manner in which supplies are purchased, controlled and distributed. The more frequent reasons given by administrators for rising supply costs are:

- poor purchasing practices such as decentralized authority and responsibility for purchasing activities, the limited role of the purchasing department, numerous rush orders and small orders and brand name preference;
- excessive inventories throughout the facility resulting from low inventory turnover, multiple storage areas and generally poor control methods;
- lack of standardization and duplication of supply items; and
- distribution methods that may not have changed with the physical growth of the facility.

Prudent purchasing can be successfully implemented by health care institutions to counteract the rise in supply costs. As an important segment of the American economy, health care providers can and should make every effort to conserve costs. Prudent purchasing procedures can lead either to saving costs or avoiding the effects of the inevitable increases we have seen in the recent past.

Spiraling costs make it imperative that all businesses undertake prudent purchasing programs. By developing a prudent purchasing program, the hospital can accomplish three important objectives.

1. It can meet the requirements of the Medicare regulations.
2. It can enhance its own financial position.
3. It can fulfill its obligation as part of the business community to reduce inflation.

REFERENCES

1. S.Rep.No. 570, 96th Cong., 1st Sess. (1979).
2. H.R.Rep.No. 2626, 96th Cong., 1st Sess. (1979).
3. Social Security Act, 42 U.S.C.
4. Social Security Act, 42 U.S.C. § 1395x(v)(1)(A).
5. 42 C.F.R. § 405.451(a).
6. 42 C.F.R. § 405.451(c)(3).
7. Medicare Prov. Reimb. Man. (CCH) ¶5858.
8. Medicare Prov. Reimb. Man. (CCH) ¶5868.

Application of the prudent buyer principle to purchasing administration

William K. Henning
Director
Management Consulting
American Hospital Supply
Division of American Hospital Supply
  Corporation
McGaw Park, Illinois

THE YEAR IS 1986. The place is a 350-bed community hospital. The purchasing administrator stops to talk to the financial director as they leave the conference room following an administrative meeting on purchasing. "Thanks again for those great computer reports," says this purchasing administrator to the financial director. "It is so much easier reporting on purchasing to the administrative staff with summary data that cover all purchases—stock purchases, routine nonstock purchases, specials. And now we have service contracts on it, too."

Several years ago, there was a flap about the prudent buyer concept. The concept was featured in a federal program as one of the obvious ways to help hospitals contain their costs. There had been the implication, much of it politically inspired, of "wasteful" purchasing practices in hospitals. After politicians had used this theme for their purposes, the prudent buyer concept became a part of the normal operating review by fiscal intermediaries.

In purchasing it had boiled down to a few basics: an audit of maximum allowable costs (from the Califano era), an audit of a "market basket" of invoice prices—all of which were known by hospitals in advance—and a simple questionnaire filled out once a year by each hospital.

The questionnaire had been embarrassing to some hospitals that had wasted valuable time waiting for the federal government to spell out the rules of its prudent buyer game. As is typical of these programs, the rules never were handed down completely: they simply evolved. And those hospitals that had not reviewed and strengthened their purchasing programs were not prepared when the initial overall program, simple as it was, started.

The purchasing administrator of the 350-bed community hospital had realized in 1979 that most of the hospital's existing purchasing procedures were quite prudent. The administrator also realized, however, that the purchasing department lacked the necessary control of *all forms* of purchasing throughout the hospital necessary to assure its personnel and someone from the outside that truly cost-conscious prudent buying was in fact being accomplished. Beyond the purchasing done outside the purchasing agent's office in pharmacy and dietary, there were some purchases initiated by the administrative offices— purchases of insurance, borrowing of money, and contracting with professionals—that needed to be pulled together in an overall control. Administration had broadened the scope of the purchasing agent's job, rewritten procedures, emphasized the work of the standardization committee and started a search for a computer capability that would (1) automatically produce the paperwork for stock purchases, (2) be the purchase order printing system for all nonstock purchases and (3) produce comprehensive monthly reports covering all forms of purchasing.

As a start, the purchasing administrator's hospital adopted the meaning of Sections 2102 and 2103 of the *Provider Reimbursement Manual,* the guide to hospital expenses that may be reimbursed for Medicare and Medicaid. The hospital developed a working definition of the prudent buyer concept: Prudent buying is the organization and administration of all forms of purchasing in the hospital applying uniform policies and procedures designed to assure cost-conscious purchasing practices within the meaning of Sections 2102 and 2103 of the *Provider Reimbursement Manual.* Purchasing is

---

Purchasing is prudent when product costs as shown on invoices and hospital costs directly related to the acquisition and use of these products—storage, distribution, processing and disposal—are the lowest that the support of quality patient care permits.

---

prudent when product costs as shown on invoices and hospital costs directly related to the acquisition and use of these products—storage, distribution, processing and disposal—are the lowest that the support of quality patient care permits.

A checklist which became the basis for the purchasing administrator's job descrip-

Table 1. Prudent buyer checklist

- Hospital policy specifying administrative approvals by dollar level.
- One uniform purchase set and one uniform policy/procedure for all hospital purchases.
- Purchase order bearing a certificate of pricing requirement: Seller warrants and certifies that prices under this order for like-quantities and like-goods shall be as low as, or lower than, those charged seller's most favored customer, in addition to any discount for payment.
- One control point for all purchasing, assuring—even for purchase orders not originated in the purchasing department—that purchasing policies and procedures have been followed.
- A purchase order covering every purchase of goods and services.
- Purchase orders numbered and issued sequentially.
- Purchase orders showing terms, prices or reference to pricing agreement.
- Comparison of quantities, prices and terms on invoices with purchase order.
- Standard specifications written for frequently purchased products. (Specifications updated periodically.)
- Establishment of Economic Order Quantities and Reorder Points for stocked products.
- Contracts specify scope of activity, terms, termination and specific price. Legal review advisable. Long-term contracts reviewed periodically.
- Nonstock purchases made upon receipt of signed requisition.
- Signature cards in purchasing for every department head authorized to requisition.
- Purchasing done in hospital departments outside of purchasing:
  - Signature card for each person authorized to purchase, indicating products or services to be purchased.
  - Blocks of purchase orders provided. Record of numbers in purchasing.
  - Design of departmental purchasing procedures by purchasing agent.
  - Adherence to system, documentation of decisions and prudence monitored by purchasing agent.
- Prudent procedures for purchasing services:
  - A written plan for the review and purchase of services.
  - Alternatives comparing quantitative and qualitative factors carefully analyzed.
  - Service provider's proposals must be related to hospital objectives and costs must be delineated in writing.
  - Proposals shall be reviewed by administration and/or trustees.
  - Reasons for purchasing decision shall be documented.
  - Contract.
- Purchasing policies to include:
  - Definition of prudent buying.
  - Conflict of interest.
  - Acceptance of gifts statements.
- Regular procedure for reviewing departmental supply expenses and inventories.
- Criteria established for vendor performance. Vendor performance monitored and an approved vendor card file maintained (updated periodically).
- Internal audits to ensure procedures are followed.
- Accounts payable rules; method of approving invoices for payment. Method for changing invoices to agree with POs.

tion and a new set of purchasing procedures was available to the hospital. (See Table 1.)

Considering the requirements in the checklist and their hospital application, the purchasing administrator's hospital administration felt they needed to formalize this purchasing effort and establish a purchasing program for the implementation of purchasing control throughout the hospital. A rather complete job description was written to provide a detailed description of the duties and responsibilities for the incumbent and to communicate the nature of the new, broad-scoped job to members of administration.

THE PURCHASING ADMINISTRATOR

Basic Function

According to the job description, the purchasing administrator reports to the assistant administrator of purchasing. As the hospital's purchasing agent, the administrator is responsible for:

- implementing and directing the hospital purchasing program to control the purchase or the lease of all goods and services from outside sources;
- purchasing, negotiating or reviewing and approving all purchase arrangements with outside sources;
- counseling and monitoring purchasing functions in other departments on behalf of administration;
- managing products in general use by establishing criteria for acceptability, cataloging, administering new product review, standardization and working with administration to ensure adequate processing and maintenance of reusable products; and
- managing the capital equipment accountability program.

Duties and Responsibilities

A. DEPARTMENTAL MANAGEMENT

The usual departmental management responsibilities.

B. ORGANIZATIONAL FUNCTION

1. Confers on a regular basis with members of administration for the purpose of coordinating the hospital purchasing program with the objectives and plans of top management.
2. Submits monthly reports concerning functional and administrative phases of the program to the assistant administrator.
3. Directs the activities of the standardization committee to assure that it meets at least monthly, is chaired by an appropriate person and that it consistently applies quality criteria and standardization principles to the products it authorizes for general use in the hospital.
4. Maintains a professional rapport with the medical staff, administration, nursing service and all other hospital departments, such that communication is adequate and the agent's expert purchasing skills are applied throughout the hospital.
5. Establishes and maintains proper and appropriate professional and ethical relationships with sales representatives and other outside contacts.

C. CENTRAL PURCHASING MANAGEMENT

1. Manages the procurement of supplies, services and equipment for and in the purchasing department.
2. As a staff person and an administration agent, controls all procurement throughout the hospital (with the exception of certain types of purchases reserved by the administrator).

3. Develops, recommends and adheres to policies and procedures relating to the management of purchasing in the hospital.

4. Abides by written hospital procedures on conflict of interest and acceptance of gifts.

5. Orders, bids, negotiates with outside sources and participates in bona fide group purchasing and shared-service efforts with other hospitals.

6. Develops and recommends to administration a purchasing system which identifies departmental personnel who should be authorized to conduct purchasing.

7. Maintains an up-to-date list of all persons in the hospital authorized to purchase from outside sources and the types of products or services they are permitted to purchase.

8. Coordinates with administration the establishment of procedures necessary for the administrative approval of purchase orders and contracts, and assures that these procedures are followed in every case within the hospital by direct supervision or by periodic auditing of purchasing activity in other departments.

9. Determines the most cost-effective and prudent method of purchase for every purchase except those reserved to the administrator. Establishes purchasing method guidelines to be followed by department heads in those departments not under the purchasing administrator's supervision.

10. Assures that an appropriately completed purchase order is issued for every purchase or group of purchases in the hospital.

11. Maintains a record of all active contracts for purchases, lease or service and a description of the type of records and location of those records not maintained and filed in the purchasing department.

12. Establishes criteria to determine which products should be made for central storage. Defines which purchases should be handled as "specials" and sent directly to departments. Reviews special purchases periodically to identify those which should be shifted from special to central distribution status within the system.

13. Reviews special requests and determines that products are completely and accurately described.

14. Shares with the distribution manager the responsibility of maintaining low inventories in the central area and throughout the hospital by means of a reliable, efficient and low-cost flow of goods from receiving to the various departments. (This is accomplished through purchasing decisions, balancing timely and reliable delivery with the costs of ordering, receiving and storing, cumulatively.)

15. For all important suppliers, establishes a method for periodically monitoring the delivery performance of each; maintains an approved vendor list.

16. Establishes simplified methods of handling repeat orders so that the process is fast, inexpensive and error free.

17. Establishes a method for identifying stockouts and quickly overcoming problems for high-volume consumables.

18. Maintains standard specifications and works with the distribution manager to establish standard purchasing quantities, reorder points (and periodically reviews these standards) for consumables within the central storage and distribution system.

19. Assures that in a department not under the purchasing administrator's control, invoice prices, quantities and terms are matched with similar information on approved purchase orders or contract forms to authorize invoices for payment and that this process is periodically audited by an outside firm.

20. Annually reviews the format and legal conditions on the standard purchase order set and updates this material with appropriate administrative and legal assistance.

21. Supervises the handling of all adjustments and claims with outside sources.

22. Engages in purchasing research and value analysis; studies market trends sufficiently to identify the lowest total-cost purchasing method forecast needs, and shares this information with appropriate hospital personnel.

D. REGULATION AND ACCREDITATION

1. Meets or exceeds standards of compliance for all accrediting and regulatory bodies.

2. Monitors all hospital purchasing to assure strict compliance with prudent buyer concepts as defined in the *Provider Reimbursement Manual.*

3. Studies the contractual requirements of hospital third-party intermediaries and determines their methods of applying the prudent buyer concept to hospital audits. Helps the hospital take appropriate action to prepare for the possibility of a prudent buyer audit.

4. Maintains files of analyses and correspondence relating to purchasing decisions such as bids, negotiations and cost benefit analyses.

5. Works with administration to establish procedures to document all prudent-purchasing actions regarding services for departmental management (such as housekeeping and dietary) and the purchase of financial packages (such as insurance and borrowing).

E. PRODUCT MANAGEMENT

1. Establishes criteria relating to quality, safety, compatibility, labeling and use-life in the case of reusable classes of products (with the assistance of appropriate department heads) for those general-use products which the hospital desires to make readily available and maintain through its materiel system.

2. Writes and assures adherence to

product and equipment specifications.

3. Reviews and makes appropriate recommendations on all new supplies and equipment, applying general hospital criteria and the considerations of standardization, cost effectiveness and other general hospital management requirements.

4. Communicates the list of products within the central system to users by means of a printed catalog or a computer system video display.

5. Manages the standardization effort primarily by guiding the standardization committee.

6. As recall coordinator assumes the responsibility of being the focal point for recalls—informing using departments, monitoring the effectiveness of action taken and maintaining all records of recall.

7. Takes appropriate action to assure that adequate maintenance is established for each of the hospital's reusable products.

8. Coordinates the necessary in-service training for new and certain existing products.

F. CAPITAL EQUIPMENT MANAGEMENT

Establishes a system which lists capital equipment by department, value and condition, assuring departmental accountability, and maintains a record for financial and legal purposes.

G. DISPOSAL OF EXCESS USABLE AND SALVAGED GOODS

1. Works with vendors and outside agencies to sell back certain excess supplies and equipment.

2. Works with outside agencies to donate certain usable goods which cannot be returned for credit and destroys the remainder (with the approval of hospital administration).

PURCHASING DEPARTMENT

A strong hospital purchasing program is founded on a strong purchasing department. The purchasing administrator uses the following guidelines to improve the methods of the purchasing department.

A. Staffing

For a 350-bed hospital in 1982 it has been assumed that there are computer programs to manage the central inventory and print stock and nonstock purchase orders, and that there is computer-terminal ordering from major suppliers.

The purchasing administrator:

- performs hospital's purchasing agent functions;
- negotiates all large agreements and contracts;
- participates in purchases of major equipment;
- establishes purchasing policies and procedures;
- reviews purchasing functions outside the department for use of the prudent buyer method and for adherence to procedure;
- directs standardization committee efforts;
- responds to recalls and hazard notification; and
- conducts in-service education programs.

The assistant purchasing agent:
- purchases nonstock products, supervises terminal and telephone ordering;
- follows up on back orders;
- monitors vendor performance; and
- assumes position of purchasing agent in the absence of the purchasing administrator.

The secretary/buyer:
- performs secretarial duties;
- operates terminal for purchase-order production and direct-supply ordering; and
- follows up on back orders with prime supplier representatives.

The equipment management program coordinator:
- monitors administrative purchase authorization; and
- maintains computer inventory of equipment location and value and maintenance record.

The additional buyer:
- may be required if purchasing department purchases pharmaceuticals and food.

B. Skillful Use of Purchasing Methods

The skillful use of purchasing methods includes the following:
- use of formal bidding of equipment and groups of items as appropriate;
- negotiation of systems contracts for routine purchases and other contracts and leases;
- employment of group purchasing where the price and services are advantageous;
- use of informal shopping (documented) on purchases that do not fit the above categories; and
- use of purchase decisions based on total cost and then documented.

C. Use of the Standard System

There is strong emphasis in the hospital on the use of the standard system—those products in the catalog, stored or handled on a routine basis by purchasing and distribution:
- use of exchange cart or parlevel systems;
- use of preprinted requisitions, catalog revised once each quarter;
- effective use of the standardization committee;
- educating "users" and assisting them in organizing their purchase requests and follow-up procedures and files; and
- refusing some special purchases requests (with administrative backing).

D. Rapport

The administrator establishes good rapport with physicians, nurses and department heads and assists them with supply problems.

E. Use of Purchasing Indices

In addition to the computer reports for inventory purchasing management:
- purchasing department expense divided by total purchases;
- purchasing department expense per patient day; and
- stock and nonstock purchases per patient day.

This model has been a projection three years into the future based on observed conditions and trends in the health field, and offers purchasing agents an initial set of goals. Today's agents need to set specific objectives and develop strategies and tactics to achieve these objectives. This look into the future pictures something more than a hospital living with the requirements of prudent buying. It describes the establishment of good business management practices for hospital purchasing and the evolution of the typical purchasing agent's job into a broader purchasing administration responsibility.

The effects of the prudent buyer concept on the supplier

Max H. Goodloe
Chairman
Whittaker/General Medical Corporation
Richmond, Virginia

HOSPITAL COST containment is a subject that has attracted the attention and interest of the entire nation. Inflation is the number one enemy, and, according to the present administration, health care providers are some of the greatest culprits. The Carter Administration has repeatedly proposed cost-containment legislation that, if enacted, would have a profound impact on the hospital industry. Although at present the containment of costs in health care institutions has for the most part been left to the voluntary efforts of individual hospitals, the government is becoming involved in hospital cost containment through the concept of prudent buying. An evaluation of the "prudent buyer" concept is valuable both for hospital materiel managers and for hospital suppliers as they face the overall problems of hospital cost containment, government intervention, and the impact of these on the relationships among manufacturers, suppliers and health care providers.

In the Medicare Procedures Bulletin number 26, the prudent buyer policy is stated as follows: "The prudent and cost conscious buyer not only refuses to pay more than the going price for an item or service, but he also seeks to economize by minimizing cost." In theory, the prudent buyer concept presents no problem for either the hospital materiel manager or for the health care supplier. What conscientious materiel manager or purchasing agent would approve of purchasing equipment, supplies, or services at a rate above their fair market value? Likewise, the health care supplier who is committed to the free-enterprise system knows that the law of supply and demand will create an environment in which the health care provider should not have to pay more than fair market value for these supplies and services. In moving from the theoretical realm to the real world, however, the prudent buyer concept appears to become more ambiguous as a guide for the hospital purchasing process. This uncertainty inevitably has a tremendous impact on the supplier. To better understand the problems and uncertainty created, it is necessary to examine the concept as it is administered, the various interpretations of this concept by the health care providers, and the effects of these interpretations on health care suppliers.

DETERMINING REASONABLE COSTS

The prudent buyer concept essentially holds the Medicare intermediaries responsible, through their auditors, for verifying that health care providers have not paid more than the "going rate" for the equipment, supplies, and services they have purchased. Should the intermediary auditors determine that a hospital has paid above the going rate for such items, they may retroactively disallow the reimbursement of these costs. If exercised, this authority could jeopardize the financial stability of a hospital. The burden of proof as to whether or not costs are reasonable and prudent lies with the hospital, and since Medicare-Medicaid audits occur after the fact, the health care provider must document and support the prices paid for purchases as reasonable costs.[1]

How then do hospitals ascertain that each item they buy is purchased at or below the going rate? How is the going rate determined? There are several purchasing philosophies currently followed by health care providers in defending themselves as prudent buyers, each of which has a unique effect on health care suppliers. The three primary philosophies currently in practice are volume (group) purchasing, competitive (bid) purchasing, and prime vendor utilization.

GROUP PURCHASING

Volume or group purchasing refers to the formation of purchasing groups to maximize the reduction in invoice costs of goods and services through volume purchasing power. In addition to the voluntary purchasing groups formed by independent, nonprofit hospitals, proprietary hospital chains also utilize their volume purchasing power to maximize prudent buying. It should be noted that there are important differences in the way in which the chains implement this volume purchasing power.

Effect on Hospitals

In theory, the main advantage that volume purchasing offers the individual hospital is a reduction in the cost of those goods and services for which the group has a contract. In practice, this advantage is most pronounced for smaller hospitals that lack any appreciable purchasing power on their own. Group purchasing has a number of disadvantages, however, that discourage many group members from adhering strictly to group purchasing contracts. Group purchasing tends to limit the flexibility of the individual member hospitals. The staffs of member hospitals may prefer a brand of product other than that available on the contract awarded by the purchasing group, or the purchasing group may not have purchasing contracts for many of the goods and services needed by member hospitals. In addition, the member hospitals may feel that the service level of the supplier to whom the purchasing contract has been awarded is inferior and on that basis justify purchasing from an outside supplier.

For these reasons among others, many purchasing groups have not realized their full potential in cost reduction because they have been unable to maximize their volume purchasing power. Even the proprietary groups, those that should be and generally are the most effective because of their direct ownership, have experienced problems with compliance to contracts. An additional disadvantage of group purchasing, often overlooked, is the fee paid by the member hospital to belong to the group. In many cases the fee paid is not offset by any cost savings.

Effect on Suppliers

From the supplier's viewpoint, there seem to be few advantages to group purchasing except in those rare cases in which both sides benefit. Theoretically, suppliers should have the majority of the business after being awarded group purchasing contracts and should be able to develop more efficient ways of handling this business to reduce servicing costs on the contractual business. In practice however this is not always possible because hospitals tend to buy outside of contracts, and because many groups are unaware that in order to receive a better price they must also try to help the vendors reduce their costs of doing business. In many instances, the same service demands that were present before the hospital joined a group persist.

Another disadvantage of the group purchasing concept to the supplier is that it places heavy competitive pressure on the distributor's already thin margins. Group contracts tend to be an all-or-nothing proposition for the supplier. Out of fear of what would happen if they ended up with nothing, many suppliers bid on group contracts at rates below their real costs of handling the business and carrying the inventory and accounts receivable. For this reason, many health care distributors, from small local independents to the regional and national chains, are receiving a less than satisfactory return on their investment. These thin margins lead directly to the ultimate disadvantage, reduced service, at the hospital level, thereby compromising the quality of health care.

Has group purchasing reduced hospitals' costs on the supplies, equipment, and services they purchase through the group contracts, thereby enabling them to meet the requirements of the prudent buyer concept? In a study prepared by the General Accounting Office (GAO) on hospital purchasing that was released in April 1979, the GAO indicated that it could find no conclusive evidence that group purchasing has enabled hospitals to obtain goods and services at lower than

The evidence seems to indicate that group purchasing does not work to the long-range benefit of the health care provider.

nongroup prices. In some instances prices paid by group hospitals were lower while in others they were higher. The evidence seems to indicate that group purchasing neither works to the long-range benefit of the health care provider, nor is it the most effective tool available to contain costs and realize the prudent buyer concept.[2]

COMPETITIVE PURCHASING

Competitive or bid purchasing is similar to volume purchasing in that purchases of supplies, equipment, and services are put out for bid to appropriate suppliers of these goods and services. Generally, the lowest bidder with an acceptable product and level of service is awarded a contract for supplying the particular item for a

specified period of time. Like group purchasing, competitive purchasing places supplier against supplier in a competitive atmosphere to ensure that the hospital will not pay more than the going rate for an item or service and will thereby guarantee the hospital's compliance with the prudent buyer concept. In general, hospitals that successfully utilize bid purchasing are larger institutions with sufficient purchasing power independent of a purchasing group. Because they do not have to conform to a purchasing group, hospitals using competitive purchasing have more flexibility than group hospitals and are thus able to avoid many of the situations that cause group hospitals to purchase outside their contracts. The major disadvantage of competitive purchasing is that its effectiveness is limited to larger health care institutions with independent volume purchasing power.

From the supplier's standpoint, competitive purchasing, like group purchasing, puts the primary burden of price competition on the distributor's shoulders. Although suppliers should not and generally do not mind this, the price reductions achieved are often minimal. Since the distributor's margin of profit is limited to begin with, the primary effect is to weaken the suppliers and to reduce the level of service they are capable of providing.

Has competitive purchasing been effective in accomplishing the concept of prudent buying in hospitals? In its April 1979 study of hospital purchasing, the GAO found that competitive bidding allowed hospitals a wider choice of supplies and products, leading to higher quality goods and services at lower prices. However, it also found that competitive purchasing was not maximized by many hospitals because of the lack of standardization of products used by hospitals due to multiple brand preferences of medical and nursing staffs, and the use of group purchasing agreements.[3]

PRIME VENDOR UTILIZATION

The use of prime vendors in purchasing and materiel management has become more widespread over the past several years. It seems to make sense to more and more hospitals to limit the number of vendors with which they do business. Like the advocates of the other purchasing philosophies, proponents of this method also claim that it helps them meet the requirements of prudent buying. However, the prime vendor principle differs fundamentally from group and competitive purchasing in the way that it attempts to accomplish prudent buying. The prime vendor in a sense becomes a partner with the hospital in its effort to reduce health care costs. Prime vendor services should provide the hospital a number of benefits, such as assurance of competitive costs through acceptance of fair profit margins and assistance in negotiations with manufacturers in behalf of the hospitals, including price protection; simplification of ordering procedure; and reduction of inventories.

How then is the prime vendor concept able to increase price competition and maximize price reductions for the hospital? By aligning itself with one supplier, a hospital enables its supplier to work with it closely to strengthen product evaluation and standardization, and to encourage and increase the use of generic products within the hospital.

Has the prime vendor concept been successful in reducing the overall costs of goods and services to hospitals? According to a GAO study released in November 1979 that was prepared for Sen. Herman Talmadge, Chairman of the Senate Finance Health Subcommittee, hospitals participating in prime vendor programs tended to have a higher cost of goods and services than did those using group or competitive purchasing.[4] These higher costs can be offset, however, by lower administrative (purchasing) costs; reduced inventory (carrying) costs; a higher level of service (fewer backorders); and other services, such as materiel usage reports.

Obviously, the potential of the prime vendor concept to reduce the hospital's total costs of the goods and services it purchases has not yet been fully realized. But this approach has much to offer the industry and should be explored in any way possible. There are many variations of this principle, and a hospital might have more than one vendor serving as its primary source so that competition can still be a factor.

EVALUATION OF PRUDENT BUYING

An evaluation of the effectiveness of the prudent buyer concept in reducing the cost of the goods and services purchased by hospitals shows that the results have been less than outstanding. Both studies of hospital purchasing completed by the GAO during the past year show that there is a high degree of inconsistency in the prices paid by hospitals for the goods and services they purchase. Although it would be impossible to place the blame for this situation on a single factor, certainly a large part of the problem lies in the fact that the prudent buyer concept has been shrouded in uncertainty and confusion ever since it was introduced. Unfortunately, with increasing pressure being applied by the administration, Congress, and the general public for the containment of health care costs, the handwriting appears to be on the wall: The future holds an increase in direct governmental involvement in hospital purchasing practices. Experience shows that increased government involvement will not only fail to achieve reduced purchasing costs but also will add another layer of bureaucratic administration that will inevitably have the effect of raising the costs of these goods and services.

How should suppliers then go about helping health care providers achieve the goal of prudent buying that the government, hospitals, suppliers, and general public all agree on in theory? How can this theory be put into practice without direct government intervention? The answer is not as elusive as one might think. If hospital materiel managers understand what Dean Ammer refers to as the "imperfect competition" that exists in the field of health care distribution and use this knowledge to be informed consumers or prudent buyers, then the free enterprise system can do what it does best: create an effective and efficient means of distribution, delivering the highest quality products and services at the lowest possible costs.[5]

A key element in accomplishing this is for hospital materiel managers to understand the nature of competition in the health care field and to use this knowledge to shift the primary price competition from suppliers to manufacturers. This shift can be accomplished by distinguishing between real and imagined brand differen-

> *The hospital should strive through strengthened product evaluation and standardization committees to eliminate* imagined *brand preference throughout the organization.*

tiation so that products can be evaluated on a comparative basis. The hospital should strive through strengthened product evaluation and standardization committees to eliminate *imagined* brand preference throughout the organization. This will allow more product standardization in the hospital and will also lead to the increased use of generic products. Both of these practices will lead to increased price competition among manufacturers, which in turn will lead to a lower cost for the hospital. Also, new efforts must be made in the industry to avoid the use of overly sophisticated and costly products by evaluating the most appropriate product for the task at hand.

In addition to developing a system for determining real product differentiation and product usage, hospital materiel managers also need to develop a system for measuring and evaluating the service level of the supplier. This system will enable the hospital to compare competing suppliers with different service levels.

Obviously a supplier who delivers a high percentage of products ordered in a prompt and efficient manner enables the hospital to reduce its costs, and this cost savings should be quantified and considered when comparing prices between suppliers. By balancing price competition between manufacturers based on quality of product and between suppliers based on quality of service, the hospital will be able to obtain maximum quality for the minimum price.

If the confusion that has surrounded the prudent buyer concept is an indication of what can be expected if the federal government should attempt direct involvement in the regulation of hospital cost containment, it is well to take warning. More regulation is not the answer. The prudent buyer principle should be either clarified or eliminated. Hospital materiel management will adhere to the theory of the prudent buyer with or without the threat of retroactive disallowance of Medicare reimbursement. The best solution is to let the free enterprise system function unhindered by the nightmare of mass regulation. Hospitals, through their voluntary effort programs, need to balance competition and cooperation with their suppliers for the achievement of their mutual goals. By standardizing products, by eliminating "imagined" brand preference, and by utilizing more generic products, real cost savings can be achieved. By developing a system for measuring and evaluating both quality of product (from the manufacturer) and quality of service (from the supplier), the hospital can truly function as a prudent buyer to ensure the purchase of maximum quality for minimum price.

REFERENCES

1. Texas Hospital Association Statewide Hospital Productivity Center. *Cheaper by the Dozen? A Hospital Guide to Group Purchasing* (Austin, Tex.: Texas Hospital Association 1979) p. 103-107.

2. "GAO: Insurers Should Tally Prices, Monitor Purchases." *Purchasing Administration* 3:10 (November/December 1979) p. 1-2, 26.

3. "GAO Hospital Purchasing Study." *Surgical Business* 42:10 (October 1979) p. 26-28.

4. "GAO: Insurers Should Tally Prices, Monitor Purchases."

5. Ammer, D. S. *Hospital Materials Management: Neglect and Inefficiency Promote High Costs of Care* (Boston: Bureau of Business and Economic Research, Northeastern University 1974) p. 69-83.

Hospital procurement and illegal price discrimination

Michael K. Gire, J.D.
Attorney
Bricker & Eckler
Columbus, Ohio

THERE WAS A TIME when nonprofit hospitals were able to provide their services to the public relatively free from the many restrictions, regulations and liabilities which plague for-profit commercial businesses. More recently, however, there has been a gradual erosion of the special status which was once enjoyed by nonprofit hospitals. Increasingly, nonprofit hospitals are being named as defendants in lawsuits because the protective barriers of charitable and sovereign immunity are no longer available in many states; and since enactment of the Medicare and Medicaid programs, nonprofit hospitals have also become targets of increased state and federal regulatory activity. To add to the problems facing hospital administrators, a new trend is developing in the area of health law which may ultimately impact upon the structure of health care delivery in this country: the federal antitrust laws.

Although the federal antitrust laws have been in existence since enactment of the

Sherman Act in 1890, it is only within the last few years that there has been any significant antitrust activity in the health care field. To date, most antitrust actions related to health care have been directed against professional organizations and insurance companies.[1,2] In two recent decisions, however, the U.S. Supreme Court has indicated that nonprofit hospitals may also be subject to the federal antitrust laws. In one of these decisions, the Supreme Court held that the activities of a local nonprofit hospital may have the requisite effect upon interstate commerce to make the hospital subject to the Sherman Act.[3] In the other decision, *Abbott Laboratories v. Portland Retail Druggists Association, Inc.*[4] the Supreme Court held that there are limitations upon the exemption granted to nonprofit hospitals from the price discrimination provisions of the Robinson-Patman Act.

THE ROBINSON-PATMAN ACT

Beginning with the enactment of the Sherman Act in 1890, the federal antitrust laws have evolved to prohibit a variety of anticompetitive trade practices. The basic federal antitrust laws today are contained in four legislative enactments:

1. the Sherman Act (monopolies and combinations in restraint of trade);
2. the Federal Trade Commission Act (unfair methods of competition and unfair or deceptive acts or practices);
3. the Clayton Act (price discrimination, acquisition and mergers, interlocking directorates, and restrictive selling and leasing practices) and
4. the Robinson-Patman Act (price discrimination).

It was the prohibition against price discrimination in Robinson-Patman which prompted the litigation leading to the Supreme Court's decision in *Abbott*.

The Robinson-Patman Act was enacted in 1936 in response to the rising concern over the growth of large retail organizations that were able to use their bargaining power to obtain price concessions from manufacturers and wholesalers which were unavailable to the small independent merchants. These favorable price concessions not only gave an unfair competitive advantage to large retailers by permitting them to purchase goods below the costs paid by their competitors; they also caused

---

This increase in costs to smaller purchasers created a competitive situation in which the very existence of the small independent merchant was threatened.

---

manufacturers and wholesalers to raise the prices charged to other customers to recover the cost of the price discounts given to the large retailer. This increase in costs to smaller purchasers created a competitive situation in which the very existence of the small independent merchant was threatened. As the Committee on the Judiciary noted in its report to the House on the Patman bill:

> ... the evidence is overwhelming that price discrimination practices exist to such an extent that the survival of independent merchants, manufacturers, and other businessmen is seriously imperiled....[5]

Thus the Robinson-Patman Act was enacted, in Congressman Patman's words, "to protect the independent merchant, the public whom he serves, and the manufacturer from whom he buys from exploitation by the chain competitor."[6]

The heart of the price discrimination provisions of the Robinson-Patman Act is contained in its first section, which amended Section 2 of the Clayton Act.[7] Under this section, it is unlawful for a seller engaged in commerce to discriminate—either directly or indirectly—in price on commodities of like grade and quality between different customers, when the discrimination has a proscribed adverse effect on competition.[8] The prohibition is applicable to any price differential in favor of one purchaser over another except to the extent that such price differential—

1. is necessary to meet the price of a competitor of the seller;
2. merely reflects the cost savings to the seller arising from the differences in the cost of manufacture, sale or delivery resulting from the differing methods or quantities in which the commodities are sold (e.g., quantity discounts); or
3. is due to changing market conditions or the marketability of the product.[9]

In addition to the basic prohibitions against price discrimination contained in Section 1 of the act,[10] there are prohibitions against certain brokerage fees and commissions,[11] certain arrangements as to merchandising services or facilities[12] and a general prohibition making it unlawful for a purchaser of goods knowingly to induce or receive a direct or indirect discrimination in price.[13] The Robinson-Patman Act also makes it a criminal offense punishable by a fine or imprisonment, or both, for persons engaged in commerce "to be a party to" or to "assist in" any transaction that to their knowledge discriminates against competitors of the purchaser of goods of like grade, quality and quantity.[14]

When originally enacted, the Robinson-Patman Act did not provide for an exclusion for charitable organizations. To remedy this situation, the Congress in 1938 enacted the Nonprofit Institutions Act.[15] This legislation granted to schools, colleges, universities, public libraries, churches, hospitals and charitable institutions not operated for profit an exemption from the provisions of the Robinson-Patman Act to the extent that these organizations purchased supplies *for their own use*.[16] The purpose of this exemption was, " ... to make certain that favors in price which are occasionally extended to eleemosynary institutions, because of the character of the institution, do not fall under the ban of the act."[17] Although the Nonprofit Institutions Act did not define the phrase "for their own use," the exemption was apparently considered broad enough to cover most purchases by eleemosynary organizations. From 1938 until the *Abbott* decision, only two reported cases challenged sales to eleemosynary organizations under the Robinson-Patman Act,[18] and in only one of these cases did the court find that the exemption did not apply.[19]

ABBOTT LABORATORIES V. PORTLAND RETAIL DRUGGISTS ASSOCIATION, INC.

The litigation in *Abbott* was instituted by a group of more than 60 retail pharmacists[20] against 12 manufacturers of pharmaceutical products (including Abbott Laboratories). The plaintiff pharmacists claimed that the defendant pharmaceutical companies had violated the Robinson-Patman Act by selling drugs to certain nonprofit hospitals—each of which had a pharmacy—at prices that were lower than the prices the pharmaceutical companies charged retail pharmacists. Both the plaintiffs and the defendants agreed that the Robinson-Patman Act would apply to this situation but for the exemption granted to hospitals under the Nonprofit Institutions Act of 1938. Therefore the issue presented to the U.S. Supreme Court for decision was: What constitutes purchases for a hospital's "own use" for purposes of the exemption from the prohibition against price discrimination granted in the Nonprofit Institutions Act?

To analyze what constitutes a purchase for a hospital's "own use," the Supreme Court placed the sales and dispensation of pharmaceutical products into the following categories:

1. to the inpatient for use in the patient's treatment at the hospital;
2. to the patient admitted to the hospital's emergency facility for use in the patient's treatment there;
3. to the outpatient for personal use on the hospital premises;
4. to the inpatient, or to the emergency facility patient, upon the patient's discharge for the patient's personal use away from the premises;
5. to the outpatient for personal use away from the premises;
6. to the former patient, by way of a renewal of a prescription given while an inpatient, an emergency facility patient, or an outpatient;
7. to the hospital's employee or student for personal use or for the use of a dependent;
8. to the physician who is a member of the hospital's staff, but who is not its employee, for personal use or for the use of a dependent;
9. to the physician, who is a member of the hospital's staff, for dispensation in the course of the physician's private practice away from the hospital; and
10. to the walk-in customer who is not a patient of the hospital.

The plaintiffs and the defendants agreed that the first three categories were purchases for a hospital's "own use," but disagreed about the remaining categories. The plaintiffs argued that the exemption should be limited to the first three categories because sales in the other categories placed the hospitals' pharmacies in direct competition with retail pharmacists. The defendants responded that the exemption should focus on the nonprofit character of the institution and should be liberally construed. Ultimately, the Supreme Court adopted a position between those urged by the parties.

The focus of the Supreme Court's analysis was neither the "competitive effect" approach urged by the pharmacists nor the "nature of the institution" approach urged

---

The focus of the Supreme Court's analysis in Abbott *was neither the "competitive effect" approach urged by the pharmacists nor the "nature of the institution" approach urged by the pharmaceutical companies.*

by the pharmaceutical companies. Rather, the Supreme Court chose to focus on whether the pharmaceuticals were to be used "... *by the hospital* in the sense that such use is a part of and promotes the hospital's intended institutional operation in the care of persons who are its patients."[21] On this basis, in addition to the first three categories noted above, the Supreme Court concluded that:

1. Categories four and five are within the hospital's "own use" because this is a continuation of the hospital care and a part of the transition from hospital care to home care.

2. Category six is not within a hospital's "own use" because the connection with the hospital has become attenuated at the refill stage.

3. Categories seven and eight are within a hospital's "own use" because the employees and physicians at a hospital are intimately related to the hospital's function. The court noted, however, that dispensation of pharmaceuticals to a nondependent family member of an employee or physician would not be for the hospital's "own use."

4. Category nine is not within a hospital's "own use" because a physician's private practice unconnected with a hospital is too attenuated to be attributed to the hospital's "own use."

5. Category ten is not within a hospital's "own use" because this is unrelated to a hospital's function, and the hospital is acting as a commercial pharmacy with respect to competing commercial enterprises.

In reaching its conclusion as to the various categories, the Supreme Court emphasized that the exemption granted in the Nonprofit Institutions Act is limited, and a hospital is not exempt from the Robinson-Patman Act merely because it is a nonprofit institution. The Supreme Court concluded, therefore, that pharmaceutical sales within categories six, nine and ten are not covered by the Nonprofit Institutions Act exemption, and are subject to a claim of price discrimination under the Robinson-Patman Act.

IMPACT OF THE *ABBOTT* DECISION

While the *Abbott* decision relates only to the sale of pharmaceuticals, the principles set forth by the Supreme Court have a general application to the exemption granted under the Nonprofit Institutions Act. The Court made it clear that hospitals (and other eleemosynary organizations) do not have a blanket exemption from the price discrimination prohibitions of the Robinson-Patman Act. If a hospital is receiving a "hospital discount," "charitable discount," or other price concession from a manufacturer or wholesaler that is greater than the price discount available to retail merchants, exemption from the Robinson-Patman Act is only available if the commodity purchased is a "part of and promotes the hospital's intended institutional operation in care of persons who are its patients."[22]

In the case of hospital pharmacies, the Supreme Court held in *Abbott* that the exemption does not apply to pharmaceuticals purchased for resale to "walk-in" customers, physicians for use in their private practices, or refill of former patients' prescriptions. Beyond pharmaceuticals, however, other hospital activities may also fall outside the "own use" exemption of the Nonprofit Institutions Act. For example, if a hospital-owned and -operated gift shop purchases merchandise for resale at a discount price that is lower than the price which retail merchants must pay for the same commodities, then, arguably, this would be a violation of the Robinson-Patman Act because the operation of the gift shop is not related to the hospital's care of persons who are its patients.[23]

In the final analysis, any activity which a hospital engages in that is not functionally related to the care and treatment of its patients, and which places the hospital in competition with a retail merchant, may be subject to a complaint under the Robinson-Patman Act if the hospital receives a discount in price that is unavailable to retail merchants. And, if a court decides that a hospital has violated the Robinson-Patman Act, the penalties can be harsh,

including the payment of three times the amount of damages suffered by the successful plaintiff.[24] The violator can also be subject to criminal sanctions.[25]

As a practical matter, the *Abbott* decision should not be the cause of any sleepless nights for the hospital administrator. It would be prudent, however, for administrators to review those operations of the hospital that are not functionally related to the care and treatment of patients, and to ascertain whether the hospital is receiving any special discounts in its purchases which are not available to retail merchants generally. If the hospital is receiving a price from a manufacturer or wholesaler that discriminates in the hospital's favor on commodities which are not purchased for the hospital's "own use," and if this discriminatory price may have more than a *de minimus* impact upon competitors,[26] then, to avoid potential liability under the Robinson-Patman Act, the hospital should discontinue the special discount.

REFERENCES

1. E.g., United States Dental Institute v. American Association of Orthodontics, 393 F. Supp. 565 (E.D. Ill. 1975); United States v. Illinois Podiatry Society, Inc., 1977-2 Trade Cos. ¶61,767 (D.C. Ill. 1977); American Society of Anesthesiologists, (FTC Dkt. No. C-2952, 44 Fed. Reg. 11060, February 27, 1979); Indiana Dental Association (FTC File No. 781-0023, 42 Fed. Reg. 53767, November 17, 1978); California Medical Association (FTC File No. 771-0005; 43 Fed. Reg. 11709, March 21, 1978).
2. E.g., St. Paul Fire & Home Insurance Co. v. Barry, _____ U.S. _____, 98 S. Ct. 2923, 57 L. Ed.2d 932 (1978); Medical Service Corp. of Spokane County (FTC File No. 761 0051), CCH Trade Regulation Reporter ¶21,195.
3. Hospital Building Company v. Trustees of the Rex Hospital, 425 U.S. 738 (1976).
4. 425 U.S. 1 (1976).
5. H.R. Rep. No. 2887, 74 Cong., 2d Sess., 4(1936).

6. 79 Cong. Rec. 9078.
7. 15 U.S.C. ¶13(a).
8. Ibid.
9. 15 U.S.C. §13(a) and (b).
10. 15 U.S.C. §13(a).
11. 15 U.S.C. §13(c).
12. 15 U.S.C. §13(d) and (e).
13. 15 U.S.C. §13(f).
14. 15 U.S.C. §13a.
15. 15 U.S.C. §13c.
16. Ibid.
17. H.R. Rep. No. 2161, 75 Cong. 3d Sess., (1938).
18. Logan Lanes, Inc. v. Brunswick Corporation, 378 F. 2d 212 (9th Cir. 1967), cert. den. 389 U.S. 898 (1967); Student Book Company v. Washington Law Book Company, 232 F. 2d 49 (D.C. Cir. 1955), cert. den. 350 U.S. 988 (1956).
19. Student Book Company, supra.
20. After the lawsuit was instituted, the plaintiffs

assigned their claims to their professional association, the Portland Retail Druggists Association, Inc.

21. 425 U.S., at 14.
22. Ibid.
23. The operation of a gift shop by a hospital is not unlike the operation of a bookstore by a university because both are offered as a convenience, but are not necessary to the purpose of the institution. In Student Book Company, supra, it was noted that self-sustaining campus book stores—where the books sold are not for the use of the universities but for resale at a profit—are not covered by the exemption of the Nonprofit Institutions Act of 1938.
24. 15 U.S.C. §15.
25. 15 U.S.C. §13a.
26. 425 U.S., at 18.

The prime supplier contract: getting the most for the hospital's supply dollar

Charles E. Housley
Associate Administrator
Saint Anthony Hospital
Columbus, Ohio

PERHAPS the most misunderstood principle in hospital materiel management today is that of the prime supplier. The prime supplier concept is based upon purchasing entire supply categories from one vendor. It is the best way to negotiate the hospital's supply dollar and represents one of the best cost-containment ideas available to the hospital. By negotiating total supply categories on an annual volume basis, the effective materiel manager can actually reduce total supply purchase price by 10 to 18 percent. For example, a hospital with $1 million volume of medical-surgical supplies can actually save $100,000 to $180,000 over its present supply cost—certainly an amount not to be taken lightly.

RESISTANCE TO THE PRIME SUPPLIER CONCEPT

However, with all of this potential, the prime supplier concept has mostly fallen on deaf ears. Even with those hospitals that now pretend to practice the concept, results have not been dramatic. Why? First of all, to most administrators, materiel managers and purchasing agents, the prime supplier technique represents "putting all your eggs in one basket." It might be asked: Is there any other way to gather eggs? Certainly to gather 12 eggs one would never consider using 12 baskets! But most hospitals use 12 or more vendors to service their medical-surgical supply needs. Mark Twain, in *Pudd'nhead Wilson's Calendar,* suggested: "Put all your eggs in one basket and—WATCH THE BASKET." This not only represents good supply sense; it represents good practice.

Second, most materiel managers and purchasing agents seem threatened by the prime supplier concept. They believe it will result in an erosion of their purchasing power and prerogative. This notion must be destroyed before it ruins the entire institution of hospital purchasing. Purchasing must be viewed only as a small function of the myriad of functions constituting the materiel management continuum, rather than as a profession. Purchasing, to be effective, must be portrayed as a function that can be mechanized for best results. Purchasing should never be confused with the art of negotiation. Negotiation is a management skill and profession, but purchasing is merely the act of using and drawing from the results of negotiation. If purchasing is taken in this context, then the materiel manager and purchasing agent will view the prime supplier concept from an entirely new perspective.

Next, the hospital materiel manager and purchasing agent perceive the prime supplier concept as limiting or restricting competition. They tend to worry about running the smaller companies out of business. The worry is groundless. If an entire business is built on the loyalty of one hospital or contract, then that business is already in serious trouble, and so is the hospital. Materiel managers also seem to feel that only the large national suppliers can compete for the prime supplier contract. However, in most regions of the country a hospital has a selection of from six to 12 candidates to consider as prime supplier. Also, the small local suppliers can effectively compete, and oftentimes get the contract.

There is also the concern that once suppliers get a contract, they will take advantage of the hospital and begin to increase the supply prices and reduce the service component. But the hospital that allows this to happen is as much to blame as is the supplier. Certain indicators should be built into any effectively negotiated prime supplier contract to prevent abuse and misuse by the supplier. Hospitals that have experimented with the concept have found that the supplier's loyalty and attention to the hospital actually increase. After all, almost any company can afford to lose $10,000 in business, but none relish the thought of losing $1 million or more. In reality, the hospital that negotiates a prime supplier contract realizes more leverage and clout over the supplier not only for price but for service and quality as well. In the long run, it is the hospital that has the advantage. By the same token, the hospital should faithfully observe the terms of the contract. In point of fact, it is more often the hospital that does not live up to the contract, rather than the supplier.

To complicate matters even more, the hospital materiel manager and purchasing agent are accustomed to bargaining for line-item prices. They are always in quest of that elusive best price for the specific supplies. They do not feel comfortable with negotiating for total dollar volume. Neither are they prepared for or comfortable with determining which deal is best in the long run—the prime supplier contract

---

To complicate matters even more, the hospital materiel manager and purchasing agent are always in quest of that elusive best price for the specific supplies.

---

or line-item bidding. For the prime supplier contract to be successful, the staff must be capable of demonstrating that in the long run the contract is best by comparing it with numbers with which the staff is comfortable: line-item extensions.

Finally, the contract represents something new. It is a departure from the past and represents new roads of endeavor. For it to become a successful replacement for proven single-line-item purchasing, it must be demonstrated that it is indeed the more economical method.

NEGOTIATING THE CONTRACT

If the prime supplier concept is the best way to negotiate for hospitals, either individually or in groups, then how can the barriers be broken down so that hospitals will accept the concept and believe in it? Hospital materiel managers and purchasing agents are accustomed to dealing with price, and any attempt to market the prime supplier concept must deal with this fundamental point. However, until now no hospital has really negotiated a results-oriented prime supplier contract. In the past what the hospitals have done is ask the various suppliers to propose a contract, and the hospitals would essentially have vendors compete with each other almost as they have in the past. This has not been successful and will not be successful because the various suppliers and vendors are not sure that the hospitals are truly interested in giving all of their supply category to them for a certain period of time.

As a result, the vendors can seem to play a game with the hospitals and may not offer them all of the benefits that the prime supplier concept really can give them. It is imperative that the materiel manager and purchasing agent decide before going into the negotiation that the hospital will stick strictly to a buying schedule with that prime supplier for a certain period of time. Vendors can be skeptical. It is likely that a hospital will not receive all the benefits of prime supplier negotiation during the first go-around. The vendor may well want first to be convinced of the hospital's commitment—and credibility—in shifting to a prime supplier system.

The Supply Priority Profile

The prime supplier contract should be built around a three-part proposal sent to suppliers. This consists of a statement of the hospital's terms, a list of major categories for prime supplier consideration and a supply priority profile. (See Appendix.) Certainly this fundamental point will address the hospital materiel manager's and purchasing agent's desire to deal with prices. The list should be the dollar volume item for that category based on priority. There should be no attempt to change brands or to standardize, and beginning the negotiations the hospital should provide the list of supplies as its past purchasing profile demonstrates. If the supplier can provide similar products at better prices in the future, so much the better.

The list of supplies should be based on Paredo's principle of 10 percent of the items taking up 80 percent of the dollar volume. Therefore, the listing should be those high-dollar-volume items that represent only a small amount of supplies and numbers, but will provide the supplier with a large annual dollar volume. The hospital should be responsible for providing such a list. This priority listing should delineate—

1. name of the item;
2. description of the item;
3. quantity to be purchased at any one time;
4. safety stock requested;
5. price protection category, which the supplier agrees to provide for the hospital.

The hospital might be well advised to provide documentation as to the quantity of these items purchased over the last purchasing year. This brings about demonstrable results. For example, the category of medical-surgical supplies would be the most encompassing and most numerous of any of the categories that will be considered under a prime supplier contract. Therefore, there will be on an average of between 350 and 500 items that will encompass the majority of the hospital's medical-surgical category. This can even be provided on a computer listing if the hospital has the inventory computerized, and it can very easily give the units and dollar volumes purchased for the past year. The hospital should provide the form and give it to each prospective prime supplier. They will in turn complete it and then return it within the specified period of time indicating their desire to enter into a prime supplier contract. There are other considerations, but the priority listing is the most important. The entire prime supplier negotiation rests upon a good supply listing with the requested information.

Delivery Time and Frequency

The hospital should request that the supplier delineate in writing a delivery time and frequency for each shipment. Frequency and means of delivery are negotiable terms—and can be very important. The hospital should build its supply priority list around a maximum that includes a delivery lead time. The prime supplier should then agree to this frequency and meet it. The hospital should try to persuade the prime supplier to provide its own source of transportation. It is difficult enough to come to terms between the hospital and the supplier without having a third party—namely, a common carrier over which neither has authority or responsibility—wedged between the two. Alternatively, the hospital may want to negotiate picking up the supplies itself from the vendor on a specified schedule. The hospital should determine the cost of such an arrangement and ask for a corresponding reduction in the overall price. The hospital should study the situation and request the one it thinks would better serve its needs.

Mode of Purchase Order Transmission

Another point of negotiation is the mode of purchase order transmission. Whatever the mode, the hospital should not pay for the use of any such input devices to the prime supplier. Many vendors have their own means of transmission of purchase data and might insist that the hospitals use it. But the hospital should have no part of it unless it is completely satisfied that such mode of purchase order transmission can be used for all of its other potential prime suppliers. The real reason that the various data transmission systems are used is to lay the burden of keypunching of all of this purchase product minutiae onto the hospital. The hospital should be aware of this pitfall and avert it during negotiations. The hospital might specify a very simple means of transmitting purchase order data to the prime vendor, a means adaptable to all of the other prime vendors. The hospital, if this concept is negotiated correctly, will probably enter into between 35 and 50 such contracts (see Appendix), so it is imperative to have a simple source of purchase data transmission.

Price Protection

Price protection is another negotiating point. There should be a checklist on the priority item listing for that specific category as to which term of price protection the supplier agrees to for each item. For example, on the priority listing there might be the numbers 1, 2, 3 and 4. One (1) should indicate price protection for three months; 2, for six months; 3, for a year; and 4, for 18 months or longer. For each of the items listed in the category the prospective prime supplier should check which price-protection term it could ensure the hospital for that item. Price protection can be worth thousands of dollars on an annual basis; it should not be considered lightly.

Penalty Clause

The penalty clause is an oft-misunderstood part of the prime supplier contract. Most hospitals feel that it is too much trouble to pick up extra cash, and some feel that the recordkeeping would be cumbersome. However, since the hospital has indicated for each of the items in the priority listing an order quantity and a safety stock quantity, these two quantities combined should represent the total quantity that the hospital could request and be assured of getting. For example, if the item were underpads and the order quantity were 25 cases and the safety stock 25 cases, then the hospital could request 50 cases of underpads and expect to receive them. If the vendor were out for any reason, barring acts of God, then the hospital would be due a direct check for a certain

The penalty clause merely ensures that the supplier will back up what he promises and will service the hospital on a priority basis.

percentage—the author recommends 5 to 10 percent—of the total dollar volume back-ordered. This serves to have the supplier back up all his claims and limits the number of back orders to almost nothing. There must be a specific delineation of the quantities to be used. These must be on file with the vendor for a period of time so that the vendor can gear up his stocking processes to accommodate such requests. After that, the vendor should produce according to the hospital's specifications and intentions during the terms of that contract. The penalty clause merely ensures that the supplier will back up what he promises and will service the hospital on a priority basis.

Price Guidelines

The hospital should del[illegible] several price guidelines for the p[illegible] supplier candidates to consider. It must remind the suppliers that they are candidates for a large volume of supply dollars. The amount should be put in writing. The hospital should ask for the best quantity price regardless of volume purchased. This simple procedure will allow the hospital to lower its inventory but still take advantage of volume buying. If, for example, the quantity price on underpads is in lots of a thousand, the hospital should get that price even though it would be expected to order only in needed quantities.

It is in the vendors' best interest to also put forth in their contracts certain supply lines that they may be able to offer at reduced prices. For instance, some of the prime suppliers may be manufacturers of their own lines, and they should indicate these by categories such as trays, instruments, etc.

Purchase Option

The contract should include an option to purchase all equipment from the contracted vendor on a prime vendor basis. This will usually take the form of cost-plus or a certain percentage off list. Price is not everything, but if the contract is to be credible, it must address itself completely and openly to price on a line-item basis.

The most accurate way for the hospital to determine which supplier has the best overall price is to take the item prices as listed by the respective vendors, multiply each by the past year's consumption and then compare the totals. Moreover, the materiel manager can compare the lowest total with the total dollar volume purchased last year to find how good a bargain has been negotiated.

Additional Price Protection

In addition to the price-protection agreements, the hospital should ask that the total costs for each year of the contract not exceed a certain percentage. Depending on the year and the rate of inflation, it would be reasonable to assume a total overall percentage of somewhere between 6 and 8 percent per year limit on the amount of increase. The vendor should also be reminded that the prices given in the supply priority listing should reflect an overall negotiated percentage off the best quantity price. He should also be required to indicate in writing what that percentage actually is. The vendor may specify this by category, and this is perfectly acceptable. Some hospitals, when negotiating the prime supplier contract, have asked the vendor to sign a statement that the prices quoted will meet the requirements of the prudent buyer legislation for hospitals. This is an absurd request for the hospital even to consider making of the supplier. The onus of prudent buyer legislation is on the hospital. It is the duty and sole responsibility of the hospital to institute a method that will gauge whether the prices negotiated meet at least a maximum allowable cost under the legislation. Before negotiating with the prime supplier, and certainly before granting the contract, the materiel manager or purchasing agent should check with several hospitals in the area to learn what prices they are paying for the contract items. The materiel manager must make every effort to determine that his or her hospital is getting the best possible prices.

Business Motivation Percentage

Another issue to negotiate with the prime vendor is the business motivation percentage. The materiel manager should have a good idea what dollar quantities the hospital will be purchasing on a yearly basis. Then the hospital should request that the prime supplier provide a motivation percentage if the business for that category reaches a certain amount. For instance, if it is reasonable that, on the basis of past experience, the medical-surgical supplies amounted to $1 million per year, then the hospital should ask that at least 1 percent be rebated if the hospital buys that amount from that dealer in that amount of time. The materiel manager may even go so far as to ask for 2 percent on $1,250,000 worth of business. Also, the materiel manager should not shrink from asking the supplier, if given the contract, to simply reduce the prices quoted by the 1 percent or 2 percent (rather than giving a year-end rebate), with the hospital agreeing to return the difference if it should fail to reach that dollar quantity. This motivates the hospital to abide by the terms of the agreement. The prime supplier contract is a two-way street and will benefit the hospital as well as the vendor—if both abide by the terms.

A materiel manager should set up a debit and credit accounting record of any offers that other vendors make during the period of the contract. If the amount of business the hospital must reach to get a rebate is $2 million, and the hospital is already taking the 1 percent in anticipation of reaching that amount, then if the hospital falls short of that volume over that period, it stands to lose $20,000. A vendor may attempt to recoup some of the business lost to the prime supplier by offering a price on sutures amounting to 1 percent off a possible $100,000 annual purchase of sutures. The materiel manager should make note of this in the debit and credit record and say to the supplier that this is certainly not enough motivation to leave the terms of the prime supplier contract. It would take an almost unrealistically large number of these kinds of lost-leader offers to even touch the contract benefits of the prime supplier contract. But the materiel manager should keep such an account—if only to show the skeptics that the contract offers the best possible advantages to the hospital.

Reports

Another consideration is that of vendor reports. The materiel manager should delineate what reports he or she feels are

---

The materiel manager should keep an account of outside offers—if only to show the skeptics that the prime supplier contract offers the best possible advantages to the hospital.

---

necessary to keep abreast of the prime supplier contract—such things as back-order reports, increased costs reports and actual volume sales. Along with the reports there should be at least a quarterly evaluation of the effectiveness of the contract. The hospital should make every effort to see that the relationship between it and vendor is on a mutually effective, results-oriented and ethical basis at all times. Reports should be of a two-way nature, with the hospital manager turning in a report on the effectiveness of the sales representative, the number of back orders, etc., and the vendor evaluating the terms of the contract in such measures as total dollar sales and increased dollar sales over past performance, etc. Another good index for the supplier to use is total dollar volume per occupied bed. This probably

should be between $1,800 and $2,400 per bed for the medical-surgical category.

Length of Contract

All contracts state the life of the contract in months or years. In the author's experience, one-year contracts are not really cost effective or performance oriented for the hospital. Some materiel managers and purchasing agents, on the other hand, feel that three years is too long a period to be committed to one supplier without testing the marketplace, so it seems that two years is a good compromise. Still, if the negotiated price protection seems far superior, a three-, four- or even five-year contract should be considered.

REQUIRED: COMMITMENT

If a hospital really practices the prime supplier concept, the total dollar volume of hospital purchasing, including supplies, drugs and equipment services can be reduced by *a minimum of* 10 percent. Some hospitals can reduce their costs by 20 percent. One can readily see that this is an excellent cost-reduction device. If a hospital has a total supply budget of $5 million and is successful in negotiating a reduction of 10 percent, this could amount to a $500,000 saving. But, once it commits itself to the prime supplier system, the hospital must stand by that commitment if it is to gain the vendor's trust—and the very real cost savings that go with it. The day has come and gone when hospital purchasing agents could divide up the spoils among several vendors and feel that they were protecting the hospital from exorbitant prices.

Statement of Terms

The objective of the hospital is to perform purchasing that will provide the Hospital with supplies that are of optimum quality accompanied by excellent service and good prices. To this end, the Hospital is proposing to purchase all or a major portion of all of the Medical-Surgical Category of supplies from a single supplier for a certain period of time, preferably two years. The Hospital is willing to participate in this method of purchasing under the following conditions.

A. *Pricing*

1. In order to be fair and considerate to all parties concerned, the Hospital has developed a brand-name list of supplies called a "Supply Priority Profile" and this Profile becomes an integral part of the proposal. The Profile of the items also delineates the quantities to be ordered and the quantities to be provided for safety stock. The Hospital will be responsible for thoroughly completing the above two columns and the Vendor will be responsible for indicating the price and price protection categories. *The Vendor is urged to complete the proposal as requested and not fragment it with other proposals.*

2. All prices quoted in the Supply Priority Profile will be at Best Quality Prices (BQP) as listed in the most current edition of the Sales Representative's Price Schedule. A copy of this Schedule will be made available to the authorized Hospital personnel.

3. In addition, all prices quoted will be at BQP less a percentage discount of _____% (unless the item is stated in the "Exceptions" category below).

4. All discounts and rebates (including the Motivation Discount) will be reflected in the unit price as stated on the invoice.

5. Furthermore, the Vendor agrees to include a Motivation Discount of _____% if this Hospital's volume annual purchases for the Medical-Surgical Category reach a minimum of $1,000,000.00. This percentage is to be reflected in the prices quoted in the Supply Priority Profile; however, if the Hospital's annual purchases do not meet or exceed the above-stated level, then at the agreed accounting period of one year, the Hospital will refund to the Vendor the stated percentage of the entire dollar volume purchased.

6. The Hospital agrees to pay all monthly invoices to the Vendor within a net 30-day period from the end of that respective month in which the invoices are incurred. (If the Vendor should give a 2%—10 days, then this should be reflected in the prices quoted under the Supply Priority Profile.)

7. If there are items or categories of items that are exceptions outside of the percentage off the BQP listed in item 3 above, please list these exceptions on a separate page under the column entitled "Exceptions to the Percentage Discount."

8. Since the Hospital agrees to purchase the majority of the Medical-Surgical Category from the Vendor, all such items are presently listed under the Supply Priority Profile. However, as items are added to this category, the Hospital will want to purchase these items from the Vendor in accordance with the above Pricing Schedule. The Hospital agrees to give the

Vendor at least 30 days' notice of such items after which the Vendor agrees to supply and keep the necessary delineated safety stock of such item or items. Such requests will be made in writing to the Vendor in the appropriate Supply Priority Profile format.

B. *Service*

1. The Vendor agrees to ship properly ordered supplies to the Hospital at least once per week through its own trucking service, FOB Hospital. The Hospital agrees to limit the number of deliveries; however, if an emergency item is needed, the Vendor agrees to expedite and deliver, FOB Hospital. The emergency situation will be kept to an absolute minimum.

2. The Vendor's sales representative will be utilized for smooth coordination of this Agreement.

3. The Vendor will provide consultation and in-service of any product or piece of equipment without charge under this Agreement as requested by the Hospital.

C. *Price Protection*

The Vendor agrees to provide price protection to the Hospital in accordance with the following schedule:

Category I. These items are price protected for at least a three-month period from the time of Agreement initiation. Any price changes must be executed at the end of a quarterly period and before the next quarter begins. In other words, there will be no price changes until the beginning of a new quarter.

Category II. These items are price protected for at least a period of six months.

Category III. These items are price protected for at least a period of twelve months.

Category IV. These items are price protected for at least a period of eighteen months.

Note: The appropriate category number should accompany each item in the Supply Priority Profile.

D. *Terms of This Agreement*

1. The terms and conditions of this Agreement shall be in effect for a period of two years.

2. The Hospital may terminate this Agreement with or without cause by giving Vendor 60 days' notice.

3. The Vendor may terminate this Agreement with or without cause by giving the Hospital 60 days' notice.

4. Prices and terms that have been negotiated previously between the Hospital and manufacturers will be honored by the Vendor.

5. If an item appearing on the Supply Priority Profile is at a much higher price than is presently being paid by the Hospital, the Hospital may delete the item from the Supply Priority Profile.

6. All deliveries from the Vendor and/or manufacturer will be FOB Hospital.

E. *Penalty Clause*

If the Hospital should order an item on the Supply Priority Profile in accordance with the quantity listed under the "Quantity of Order" and "Safety Stock," and the Vendor does not have that quantity of that item, the Vendor agrees to pay as direct credit to the Hospital the greater amount of (i) the sum of _____% of the total amount of the cost of the item not shipped directly to the Hospital, or, if the item is an emergency, (ii) the difference in cost of having to get the item from another vendor.

Since the Hospital intends to participate totally in the Prime Supplier Agreement, should the Vendor ever be out of an item and that item is needed immediately by the Hospital, then the Vendor or sales representative shall obtain that item from some other source for the Hospital.

F. *Reports*

The Vendor agrees to provide monthly reports of usage, backorders, etc., for all items purchased under this proposal and make them available on a timely basis to the Hospital.

G. *Deadline*

VENDORS' QUOTATIONS MUST BE RECEIVED NO LATER THAN 12 NOON THE _____ DAY OF _____, 19____. THE QUOTATIONS THAT ARE LATE WILL NOT BE CONSIDERED. FURTHERMORE, VENDORS WHO ALTER THIS PROPOSAL WILL STAND THE RISK OF HAVING THEIR PROPOSAL NOT BEING CONSIDERED.

Major Categories for Prime Supplier Consideration

A. Medical-Surgical
1. Medical-surgical supplies in general
2. Intravenous solutions and sets
3. Dressings
4. Cardiac and vascular implants
5. Orthopedic implants
6. Surgical instruments
7. Bulk oxygen
8. Cylinder and tank gases
9. Monitoring equipment

B. Pharmaceuticals
10. Direct drugs
11. Indirect or wholesale drugs

C. Office Supplies
12. Office supplies in general
13. Office equipment
14. Typewriters
15. Copiers
16. Paper supplies

D. Printed Matter
17. Single page forms
18. Business forms
19. Envelopes and stationery

E. Dietary supplies
20. Staples
21. Fruits and vegetables
22. Meats and poultry
23. Frozen commodities
24. Bread and bread products
25. Beverages
26. Paper products
27. Dietary disposable items
28. Silverware and utensils
29. Dietary equipment
30. Vending contracts
31. Milk and milk products

F. Maintenance
32. General supplies
33. Plumbing supplies
34. Electrical supplies
35. Heating, air conditioning, ventilation supplies and equipment
36. Biomedical engineering items

G. Linen
37. Patient care items
38. Surgical linen
39. Uniforms
40. Draperies and curtains
41. Contract laundry

H. Housekeeping
42. General housekeeping items
43. Detergents and cleaning compounds

I . Radiology
44. Film and chemicals
45. General supplies
46. Diagnostic and therapeutic equipment

J . Laboratory
47. Miscellaneous/general supplies
48. Chemicals
49. Sera
50. Blood and blood products

Supply Priority Profile

Item	Description	Order Unit	Order Quantity	Safety Stock	Unit Price	Previous Dollar Volume	Price Protection Category				
							1	2	3	4	5
1 Electrodes	Long-term, adult	each	500	1,000		$120,000					
2 Admission Kits	Made to order	each	600	1,000		99,000					
3 Sutures	Ethicon 811H	dozen	15	10		87,000					

To be completed by the Vendor

(List 350–500 medical-surgical supplies based on volume priority. For example, No. 1 is the largest dollar volume item purchased, No. 2 is the second largest dollar volume item purchased.)

Computerized purchasing, materiel management and accounts payable systems: planning, features and selection

Willard H. Rosegay, M.H.A., Pharm.D.
Health Care Finance Group
Shearson/American Express
San Francisco, California

SEVERAL TRENDS occurring in the hospital industry are responsible for the growing use of computerized systems for managing the acquisition, storage and distribution of materiel in hospitals. Prominent among these are the increasing use of cart exchange systems, shared purchasing and warehousing arrangements, and the general adoption by the hospital industry of more sophisticated business practices. These include not only effective and economical inventory management, but also improved purchasing practices, bid letting and optimal use of trade discounts.

The computer software industry has responded to this new demand with a proliferation of firms offering literally dozens of software packages from which to choose. In addition, consulting firms offer hospitals the option of developing a customized materiel management system. These customized systems may be appropriate for large hospitals or multi-institutional systems, but they are usually beyond the reach of smaller and medium-sized hospitals. Before a materiel manager can select a software package that will be effective for the hospital, the hospital's needs must be assessed, and the features available in the various packages must be studied in light of the hospital's needs.

INITIAL PLANNING

The most common misconception that exists among materiel managers is that their hospitals are too unique or their requirements too specific for any commercially available materiel management software to be suitable. All institutions have some unique needs; however, the objective of the software evaluation process is to weigh the institution's unique requirements against the cost of custom development or modification, and against the balance of the system requirements that are not unique. As often as not, an initial negative outlook on software packages is little more than a smokescreen intended to hide the department manager's concern over job security or to hide how poorly the system is presently functioning.

Importance of good manual procedures

In fact, this attitude may mean that there is a great deal wrong with the present system. As a rule, a computer will not solve the problems of a bad system. A computerized system will never be better than the procedures that control it, and a computerized system with poor procedures will simply deteriorate that much faster than a manual system with poor procedures.

The soundness of the set of procedures behind a materiel management system has ramifications in the development of a com-

If a system has good manual procedures, then the adjustments required to adapt those procedures to a computerized system are not difficult to make.

puterized system. If a system has good manual procedures, then the adjustments required to adapt those procedures to a computerized system are not difficult to make. Unfortunately, since most computerization projects are undertaken to revamp failing systems, sound procedures often do not exist, or at least are not being followed. If this is the case, then the first step in computerizing the system is to develop a set of procedures that, when followed manually, function effectively. Such procedures then provide the framework for deciding which features are needed in a software package, and thus one means for distinguishing among them.

User involvement in planning

Another tenet to recognize at the inception of the project is the need for communication with and involvement of all prospective users of the system during the development process. The importance of this involvement cannot be overstated. There are at least two reasons for this.

First, maintaining a level of awareness among prospective users prevents barriers from being thrown up at the instant the system is turned over to the users because they will be generally familiar with the system, and problems they recognized will have been solved already or at least addressed. Second, user involvement produces a wealth of practical design suggestions that might otherwise be overlooked by a team of persons without day-to-day contact with the present system. This involvement goes a long way toward ensuring acceptance of the system.

However, because of the large number of prospective users of a computerized materiel management system, direct involvement by all is not feasible. Typically, a management advisory committee (MAC) composed of involved department heads or other top-level individuals is formed. The MAC is responsible for maintaining an appropriate level of awareness among lower-level employees within their respective departments.

MAC may include the directors of materiel management, data processing, accounts payable, nursing services, dietary services, pharmacy, radiology, laboratory and maintenance. From the MAC, a smaller group of people, such as data processing, materiel management and accounting personnel, forms an executive committee to undertake the technical aspects of designing, evaluating and installing the system.

In hospitals with a shortage of technically qualified personnel, management consulting firms with expertise in systems design are useful for undertaking the work involved with systems design, development of procedures, installation, documentation and testing.

The MAC holds scheduled meetings and reports to hospital management at checkpoints identified in advance or as needed for the resolution of problems that may arise. The committee should not become dominated by an individual whose interests do not represent those of the group as a whole, or who is otherwise known for an unwillingness to compromise. For example, a purchasing director might be able to push through certain features that he or she feels are essential for the effective functioning of the purchasing department, but that create inconveniences for all other users of the system. One way to minimize the dominance of nonrepresentative viewpoints is to select an individual other than the purchasing, materiel management or accounts payable representatives to chair the group.

ASSESSMENT OF NEEDS

One of the first steps in planning a new materiel management system is deciding to what extent the system is to be integrated with other hospital systems. Usually this is not a difficult problem because the centralization of purchasing, receiving and accounts payable is accepted, and because these three areas are very interdependent for data.

Absolute centralization is effective only where individuals who previously performed parts of these functions gain confidence in the workability of the centralized system. Specialized areas that frequently produce problems of this type are pharmacy and food services. In the case of pharmacy, legal restrictions may make it illegal for a nonpharmacist to order drugs, or a nonpharmacist to receive drug shipments. In the case of food services, the dietician may prefer to purchase foodstuffs directly from a vendor's truck, completely bypassing the centralized purchasing and receiving functions. Methods must be devised which allow for the required degree of flexibility but which do not allow necessary controls to be undermined.

The logical level of integration of a materiel management system with other hospital systems is to develop a single system which can ensure that:

- goods that are requested for purchase have been duly authorized and are purchased from the hospital's established vendor;
- goods that are received were ordered;
- goods that have been invoiced were purchased and received.

This level of integration is referred to as the *three-way match,* and the resulting system is called a *three-way integrated system.* This system provides a useful framework for evaluating the available software packages and will be the choice of most hospitals. Single components of the purchasing/receiving/materiel management/accounts payable cycle are available as stand-alone packages if desired.

Computerization of a system that integrates purchasing, receiving, inventory and accounts payable must retain all the controls that would normally be present in a manual system. Purchase orders must still be created with valid purchase order numbers (although they need not be *printed* since a computer record of the number is created). Purchase requisitions must be duly authorized prior to the creation of a purchase order. Receiving personnel should not be aware of the quantities of items they expect to receive. The accounts payable function must have knowledge of the purchase and receipt of goods prior to authorizing payment. The accounts payable function must include the provision

for authorization of payment of invoices for services routinely received, such as telephone, and for services that must be verified, such as elevator maintenance.

The need for attention to controls comes mainly during the development of procedures. While the computer can prevent payment of invoices for goods not purchased or received, it cannot prevent payment of fraudulently approved invoices or invoices for which receipt data cannot be documented but that have been entered into the computer. The required controls include the creation of source documents and the separation of functions, according to the most traditional accounting standards. The function of the computer is to eliminate the need to make and send copies of documents. The source document itself must still be created.

In addition to planning for the level of integration of the system and reviewing procedures for the adequacy of controls, additional planning includes reviewing the existing system for areas of weakness and for new features that may be desirable but not required. This step includes an interview with each experienced user of the present system to solicit comments. The data gleaned from these user interviews should be thoroughly reviewed by the MAC to determine the merit of the points noted.

INITIAL SOFTWARE EVALUATION

Simultaneous with the systems definition process, individuals with technical expertise or other interested MAC personnel should begin to review the software market to identify candidate systems based on the preliminary or minimum design specifications. In addition to functional requirements, this preview should include other important factors such as:

- price of the package;
- size and age of the software vendor;
- hardware requirements;
- batch versus on-line processing mode.

It is difficult to be too careful in selecting software. Some three-way integrated systems may have all the desired functions, but may be more appropriate for a nationwide manufacturing concern than a hospital. Usually, the system's level of development is reflected in its price. Other systems have been developed for specific (nonhospital) clients, and then "generalized" for sale to other clients. Such systems can be spotted by their lack of flexibility and by their use of peculiar procedures which appear to have been designed to solve a specific problem that would never occur in hospitals, such as a system driven by a bill of goods.

The goal of the preliminary software review is to identify three truly general systems that offer all the basic system requirements and that were developed by a reputable vendor who has been in business for at least ten years. At the present time, several packages that meet the needs of hospitals are available for somewhat less than $120,000.

It is probably no longer necessary to consider the custom design of a three-way integrated materiel management system, except for the most highly specialized situations. Such development efforts are enormous undertakings and are extremely expensive. While the use of commercial packages may limit the range of desirable features, most systems on the market perform all the basic functions, and some have become quite elegant.

FEATURES OF COMPUTERIZED THREE-WAY INTEGRATED SYSTEMS

The marketplace offers prospective purchasers of computerized materiel management systems a broad range of features and complexity, ranging from $8,000 skeleton systems to comprehensive $400,000 systems. There are many features that differentiate the software which can be reasonably expected in a moderately priced system.

Batch vs. real-time

Probably the most volatile and visible issue is whether the system needs to be on-line or batch. Often, the naive impres-

---

Probably the most volatile and visible issue is whether the computerized system needs to be on-line or batch.

---

sion is that on-line means that computer terminals are conveniently located in everyone's work area. After being apprised of the true significance of these terms, adamant on-line proponents may become less so.

The terms *batch* and *on-line* refer to the method by which the data files are updated. A batch system accumulates all data entries (transactions) and then posts them to the files once per day or per cycle. Therefore, in a batch system, the data files, such as inventory levels, quantities on order or dollars invoiced, will be accurate only once per cycle, at the beginning of the cycle before the first transaction has occurred.

Sophisticated batch systems allow the files to be queried at any time via a terminal or CRT, but the data still reflect the status at the beginning of the cycle.

At the other end of the spectrum of timeliness is the real-time system in which files are updated instantaneously at the point of data entry. In such a system, an inventory clerk would (theoretically) be able to determine the exact number of an item in stock, even though there may be a dozen clerks processing inventory requisitions.

It is not possible to provide a hard-and-fast rule about the appropriateness of batch or real-time materiel management systems for hospitals, but the issues should at least be aired.

First, real-time systems are significantly more complex and costly, both in terms of the initial investment and in terms of the computing capacity required to make them operate properly. If computer capacity is limited, the hospital's long-range data processing plan may place a higher priority on a real-time patient order entry system than a real-time inventory management system. Implicit in this setting of priorities is the value of the individual's time and the value of instantaneously accurate information as opposed to the cost of alternatives. With regard to materiel management systems, accurately established reorder points, economic order quantities, and timely purchasing and restocking may allow a system to operate quite effectively with information that is always somewhat dated.

Second, real-time systems require strict data input controls and procedures. Discipline among operators is a must, and a higher level of training is required for a larger number of people. Security systems must be devised and protected so that data cannot be fraudulently or spuriously entered and so that audit trails are always left. These mechanisms include password requirements, computer files of all transactions done at each terminal in the system and restrictions as to which types of transactions may be entered at each terminal or during which part of the day.

Third, real-time systems require a rather sophisticated staff of data processing personnel to constantly monitor the system. These personnel must be available at a moment's notice should problems arise. In larger hospitals, this could mean a data processing department staffed around the clock. By contrast, a system that is updated nightly could suffer a breakdown for one cycle and no great inconvenience would occur aside from a doubling of the number of transactions to process the following cycle.

Because of the complexities and expense of real-time systems, a sort of hybrid system has been developed which retains many of the virtues of both batch and real-time systems, but which avoids many of the problems. This type of system may represent the ideal compromise of features for a hospital materiel management system. This system allows transactions to be completed on-line so that stacks of computer cards do not require nightly processing. However, the files are still updated batch-wise during nightly processing from temporary files of transactions which accumulated during the day. In such a system, the data files are still out of date throughout the cycle. Unfortunately, it is often not possible to query the transaction file either to examine a specific transaction.

In such a system, file queries or reports show the status of the system only as of the beginning of the cycle. A list of transactions that contained errors is also produced each cycle, which means that someone must trace the error and enter the transaction correctly the next cycle.

These hybrid systems with on-line transaction entry and batch file updates require many of the same strict controls that true real-time systems require, but offer the convenience of reduced document flow. In addition, they are less complex technically and offer the advantage of the efficiency of batch file updating.

Item master file

An item master file is a computer file of every item that is routinely ordered by the hospital. An item master is difficult to create, however, because all routinely purchased items must be identified and described generically and have their sources identified. Sophisticated item masters list a main vendor, such as a prime vendor, and one or more alternate vendors. An item is ordered simply by inputting its code number, and the computer then abstracts all the purchase order data required for the item from the item master, and begins to build a purchase order. At the same time that the item is ordered, the usage record for the item is updated. This allows a report of item usage by item type and vendor to be prepared for use in estimating annual volumes, budgeting and negotiating contracts for guaranteed volumes of items.

An item master file may be considered to be unnecessary for smaller hospitals because of the difficulty in setting it up and maintaining it. This would be a legitimate reason for selecting a system without an item master. However, it is a key feature in large hospitals' systems with prime vendor contracts or in shared purchasing arrangements. Some vendors maintain their own item master files to induce hospitals to purchase through them. Whenever a vendor is willing to maintain a master file and still offer competitive prices, the vendor should be given favorable consideration.

Vendor master file

Like an item master file, a vendor master file is a nearly complete list of the vendors from whom the hospital routinely purchases its supplies. The vendor master file is the source of information about the vendor that is applied automatically to the purchase order which was initiated by the vendor identification on the item master file. In addition to the vendor's address and previously agreed-upon terms, the vendor master also contains minimum dollar data which govern the size of the purchase order that may be cut by the system. At the time of creation of the purchase order, the vendor's record is updated with the dollar amount for purposes of monitoring the value of total purchases from all vendors over a given period of time.

The record also contains data about the timeliness of delivery, stockouts, damaged shipments and other statistics pertinent to the evaluation of a vendor's performance. Sophisticated systems automatically purge the vendor file of inactive vendors, or of vendors specified in advance as one-time vendors.

Purchase order creation

In systems that have both item and vendor master files, the creation of a purchase order is a simple matter of specifying the item code. The system selects the prime vendor and creates the purchase order from stored data. A system that allows purchase orders to be created so easily must have correspondingly effective controls over the process. For reorders not initiated automatically by the system from inventory data, purchase requisitions should be retained as a source document authorizing the transaction.

Control over the entry of purchase order data usually takes the form of terminal controls in on-line systems. Such controls include passwords for persons authorized to create purchase orders, logs of all transactions on each terminal, and restrictions on a terminal's permitted functions.

In batch systems, all purchase transactions must have authorized source documents, and these source documents are summarized on the batch header document. Retracing a purchase requisition is then a matter of identifying the batch number and pulling the source document from that batch. When a valid purchase order is created, its contents are also posted to an open purchase order file maintained by the system. This file then serves in subsequent steps to store information about the status of the order. At the time the purchase order is actually produced or transmitted, most systems produce some type of notification copy for the requisitioning department.

Receipt recognition

In properly controlled systems, receiving personnel have access to identifying data about items expected but not about quantities. With terminals available to receiving personnel, the temptation is to allow receipts to be entered directly into the system, without the benefit of a hardcopy receiving slip. This temptation should be resisted, even over the objections of receiving personnel, for the simple reason that data entry leaves no perceptible change in the item itself. This creates the opportunity for double counting and omissions.

Optimum use of the computer in the receiving area is again for the reduction of paper flows and the ready availability of data. By inputting the purchase order number of a receipt obtained from the shipping documents, the system can produce a receiving copy of the purchase order just as a carbon copy would serve in a manual system. This document becomes the source document for receipts. Receipt data are input to the computer by an individual who reads them from the source document, a function that could take place with equal ease in the data processing department or in the office of the receiving dock.

The computer facilitates receipt data entry by displaying a facsimile of the purchase order on the terminal screen. Receipt of the items as ordered is indicated simply by inserting an x in the appropriate box on the screen. Partial receipts are indicated by typing in the number received in the appropriate field. Only primitive systems with on-line data entry will require any additional identifying data about the item to be entered. Since the primary purpose of a computer is to store data to avoid repetitious data entry, systems that do not offer this expeditious means of receipt data entry should be eliminated from consideration.

Inventory management functions

Computerized materiel management systems offer several features beyond the basic recording of additions to and withdrawals from inventory. These include such features as storeroom network design, novel general ledger interface capabilities and automatic calculation of inventory statistics. The distinctions between avail-

---

Computerized materiel management systems offer several features beyond the basic recording of additions to and withdrawals from inventory.

---

able systems are based primarily on these more advanced features.

Storeroom network design is the procedure for optimizing control over the disposition of inventory and the collection of information related to it. For example, a single storeroom is adequate for a hospital that does not track inventory items once they leave the storeroom (presumably with a proper requisition). However, this level of control also makes it difficult to install effective controls over the capture of charges because there is no accountability for the item once it leaves the storeroom. All lost charges can be traced no further than the requisitioning unit.

Single storeroom systems will inventory or expense goods upon receipt into the storeroom and will expense or transfer charges when they leave the storeroom. Economic order quantity and reorder point calculations are based solely on activity at the storeroom level, and accordingly cause the maintenance of total inventory at a higher dollar value than a system that tracks goods further along toward their point of consumption. An example of an application of the single storeroom would be in dietary, where removal of an item from stores usually means that it will soon appear on the menu. Little useful information is gained by tracking the use of a bag of sugar.

A hierarchical system is capable of tracking inventory through a cascade of storerooms and calculating the inventory management statistics at each level, and for the system as a whole. A typical cascade of storerooms might include a warehouse, storerooms in two different facilities, sterile and nonsterile stores within a facility, and finally a cart exchange system at the lowest level. Such systems allow cart inventory to be tracked, thereby providing a means for pinpointing sources of lost charges. If carts are exchanged each shift, then lost charges can be traced to the shift.

The responsibility of the MAC group in designing a storeroom network will be to decide how closely it is useful to track supplies, taking into account how serious the lost charge problem is at the hospital and the likelihood of ensuring nurses' cooperation in entering all the data required to track supplies at the nursing unit level.

Sophisticated inventory networking systems also allow specifications to be placed on the types of items that may be received into or requisitioned from any storeroom. For example, such systems would prevent pharmaceuticals from being held in general stores and foodstuffs from being issued to nursing units. Controls such as these would be difficult to implement in systems that did not provide for the complete description of each storeroom.

In practice, a network composed of about three levels of hierarchical and parallel storehouses proves adequate. Although it is possible to bring a great degree of imagination to bear upon the design of an inventory tracking system when a computer is available, the design should be guided by the value of the information to management considered in the context of the effort required to collect it. Other issues include the value of the inventory being controlled, the degree of liability associated with it and the likelihood of its diversion.

While the storeroom network is being designed, the accounting department should remain closely involved in the design of the accompanying bookkeeping system. Each time an exchange between storerooms or an issue from a storeroom to an end user is made, a ledger entry determined by the issuing and receiving account numbers is made.

Although practices vary widely, third party reimbursement considerations usually provide the incentive to move supplies off the books as rapidly as possible. Accordingly, a system might be designed in which supplies inventoried at the top level of the hierarchy were accounted for as inventory, while all transfers at levels below the top were treated as interdepartmental transfers of charges. Thus items would be expensed as early as practical upon issue from the highest level storeroom.

In addition to inventory management statistics, computerized systems compile usage statistics for each generic item. This allows trends to be monitored and future requirements to be anticipated. These data would be useful not only for negotiating prime vendor contracts, but could also be used to identify trends in item utilization early on, thereby positioning the hospital to take advantage of current favorable prices.

Voucher creation

When accounts payable receives an invoice from a vendor, it must first be matched to the corresponding purchase order and receiver before it is approved for payment. This vouchering procedure is probably the area of greatest relief offered by a computerized system, because the system takes over the responsibility for visual scanning of the documents, matching and performing adjusting calculations. Again, because of the need for an audit trail, it is still desirable to assemble the voucher packet, but the packet is used only for audit purposes, rather than for the traditional vouchering function.

A computerized system performs the vouchering procedure in the following way. When the invoice is received, entry of the purchase order number retrieves the record of that purchase order from the open purchase order file and displays it on the screen. The number of each item invoiced, along with the unit price and extension, is entered on the preformatted line. The system then verifies that an identical number of the item was ordered and received, that the price agrees with the stored price and the terms agree with the terms that apply to that vendor, and that the extension is accurate. If there is perfect accord on all items specified (within predefined tolerance ranges) then the open purchase order record is closed out and transferred to a voucher file. All items on the voucher file theoretically are ready for payment when payment comes due.

If, on the other hand, a three-way match was not achieved, the record on the open purchase order file remains open. This allows for backorders and partial shipments to be handled while ensuring that double payment is not made. Some systems have the ability to automatically initiate a new purchase order from an alternate vendor if a purchase order issued to the prime vendor remains open, either for a specified period of time or until a minimum allowable stock level is reached. Reports of aged, open purchase orders are prepared periodically for the purpose of purging expired purchase orders from the system. Some systems will purge purchase orders automatically when they reach a certain age.

Payment processing

Once an invoice has been approved for payment by the automated three-way matching process (or manually for invoices not accompanied by receivers or purchase orders), the next area of responsibility for the computer is to determine the optimum payment time. In the case of a routine purchase order the payment interval is determined by the payment terms that exist on the vendor record. The frequency with which checks are cut may be specified by the user. The system then prints checks for all approved vouchers that have discount dates before the next check printing date. In this way, the system tracks the invoice and discount dates and prints a check as late as possible to still claim the discount.

There are many options available from software vendors for the printing of checks. These include grace days for late payment while still taking the discount, automatic discounts regardless of date and algorithms that calculate the optimal.

Because some of these options may seem somewhat heavy handed, it is important to determine exactly how each candidate system handles payments, since some systems are programmed to automatically take the heavy-handed approach. This could eliminate the hospital's ability to comply with terms that might be negotiated in the future. For example, one major accounts payable system does not have the provision to pass up the discount, regardless of date. This could necessitate many manual adjustments to the system. Generally, as many options as practical should be retained for specification by the user, and systems that are coded to preempt these options should be avoided.

Other options offered by many systems include screens related to the printing of checks, such as holding all payments to a specific vendor, or the requirement of an additional level of approval for checks over a specified dollar amount. One capability that should be given consideration is the ability to produce a report of all payments that will be made in the upcoming cycle unless some action is taken. This preview list will provide the accounts payable supervisor with a final opportunity to hold payments or otherwise review the payments to be made. The list should contain all the details that will appear on the remittance advice portion of the check, specifically, the number of each invoice covered by the check; the gross, discount and net amounts for each invoice; the date of each invoice; and the total amount of the check.

In addition to printing checks for

approved invoices, it usually will be desired to retain the ability to produce ad hoc checks for situations outside the normal procedures, such as cash advances or emergency checks. Although these occasional checks can easily be produced manually in the accounts payable department, the data relating to the payment must be entered into the system to maintain a complete record of all disbursements made. Since it may also be desirable to have the system produce a check on demand, strict controls must be maintained to prevent checks from being fraudulently produced.

Several control procedures are available to minimize the possibility of diversion of hospital assets. One of the most effective is

---

Several control procedures are available to minimize the possibility of diversion of hospital assets. One of the most effective is by using prenumbered check stock.

---

by using prenumbered check stock. Systems that accept prenumbered checks require that the first check number be input at check printing time so that the system can number its own internal records correctly. The same control procedures that applied to checks under the prior manual system then apply to the disposition of checks under the computerized system. As important as this control procedure may seem, there are several accounts payable packages that print a check number on a bank check at the time the checks are printed, thereby completely bypassing this most simple and effective control point. While this method of operation may have been easier for the developer of the

package to program, many accounts payable managers view this as an unacceptable sacrifice of control.

Check processing

When checks are cut, the system records each check number, amount, payee, date and paying bank. This file then serves as the source of comparative data against which the bank tape of cleared checks is processed. Most software vendors provide the programming effort needed to develop this simple interface in the cost of the system. By running the bank tape against the file of outstanding checks, cleared checks, checks outstanding and checks cleared in error are reported. Aside from the obvious audit value of this report, some systems produce summary statistics of clearing times by vendor, which the hospital's cash manager may find useful.

VENDOR EVALUATION

Thus far, the selection criteria for a materiel management software system have been limited to an assessment of the hospital's needs and a discussion of some available features. Of equal importance, however, is the reliability of the software vendor. The need for careful examination of the vendor's credentials arises from the profitability of the systems field and the absence of standards for judging the quality of software. As a result, a certain amount of reliance must be placed on the marketplace to filter out inferior vendors. In simple terms, this means that the acceptable candidate must have several years worth of business experience.

The preliminary software evaluation which has been under way since the early phases of the planning effort will have revealed several systems that may meet the basic requirements deemed necessary by the MAC. A more intensive evaluation of features will probably narrow the field even further, leaving three or four candidates. The detailed and complete documentation of the software should be requested from the vendors at this time. If there is any hesitation about surrendering the documentation, the vendor should be dropped from consideration. This is because the absence of readily available documentation implies that the package is not seasoned.

It is not a good idea to allow the hospital to be used as a test site for a package, because "working out the bugs" is a slow and tedious process which can jeopardize the acceptance of the system by users who may become frustrated. There are several materiel management systems already functioning in the field which have passed the test of time, and there is little reward for volunteering to reinvent the wheel.

The detailed evaluation of the software documentation should consider, at a minimum, all of the following points.

- Function. Does the system basically do everything desired?
- Sophistication. Is the system too complicated for the hospital's needs or so simple that the needs may not be met?
- Price. What is the value of the inventory being controlled and the dollar volume of purchases being made, and what is the magnitude of the potential savings compared with the price of the system?
- Ease of use. Does the system interact with users; require input on screens of

data it already has on file; use clearly formatted screens; avoid the use of long strings of digits; provide clear, concise reports at various levels of detail?
- Quality of documentation. Does the documentation answer the question, "How do I do *X*?" Is it logically organized? Is it free of signs of having been patched together? Is it concise? Is systems documentation provided? Are interface coding requirements described in detail? Are sample forms provided?
- Vendor references. How many current users are there? Established vendors may have 100 or more packages in place. Is the list of references printed formally, and is it complete? Do contacts with references reveal a consistent pattern of satisfaction? Are vendor personnel prompt about answering questions about the package, or do they always seem to have to get back to you?
- Technical issues. Is the code modular in design so that future enhancements or customization may be easily implemented? Is processing efficient? Are there adequate controls over the integrity of data and files? Are there any bottlenecks in the code? What happens when several users attempt to use the system at the same time? How much disk space and memory are required?

These questions should convey the importance of skepticism in the evaluation of a vendor and the product, but none will give a qualified vendor any difficulty. Software vendors are notorious for making unsubstantiated claims and overzealous marketing pitches. There are several things which the MAC can do to guard against being misled.

- When a vendor says that the system can do *X*, ask how.
- Demand a *complete* list of the vendor's clients.
- Contact as many clients as necessary to obtain a consensus about the vendor and product.
- Do not accept an invitation to observe the system in operation at the vendor's headquarters or at a client site arranged by the vendor.
- Arrange an on-site visit to at least one of the vendor's clients to see the system in operation. Speak to client personnel who were involved with the installation of the system.

- Negotiate a contract that provides for a major portion of the purchase price to be paid only upon the demonstrated satisfactory performance of the system.
- Above all, understand the system thoroughly.

•   •   •

The planning and organization required to identify and evaluate a computerized integrated materiel management system require time and effort. With the proper approach, a system that increases control; reduces investment in inventory, purchasing costs, and lost charges; and improves personnel morale can be successfully selected.

SUGGESTED READINGS

Powell, P.B. "Computerized Purchasing, Inventory System Developed by Humana Inc." *FAH Review* (January/February 1982) p. 50-54.

Williams, H.G. and Toole, J.E. "Evaluating and Selecting a Computer System." *Topics in Health Care Finance* 4 (Summer 1978) p. 73-91.

Pharmacy purchases can be systematized

Robert L. Siddall
Manager, Contract Operations
Detroit Medical Center Cooperative
    Services, Inc.
Detroit, Michigan

DURING THE LAST five years the health care industry has been under increasing pressure from all sides to reduce expenditures. More and more, state and federal governments and other third party payers are instituting policies that require hospitals to scrutinize their operations for ways to cut costs. This increased activity has produced a revolution in the way the business of procuring goods and services for these institutions is conducted. Materiel managers and purchasing managers are being forced to develop new techniques of cost cutting and product standardization that will lead to reduction of hospital expenditures.

The prime responsibility of a purchasing manager is to procure at the lowest price possible goods and services that are consistent with the demands of quality and need. Secondarily, the purchasing manager must ensure that good business practices are being followed and that all potential vendors are treated fairly and honestly.

PLANNING THE TAKEOVER OF PHARMACEUTICAL PURCHASING

Once a purchasing department has solidified control over procurement of general hospital supplies, the question of where else the system could be applied arises, and attention is likely to turn to the pharmacy. Assuming procurement control over pharmaceutical supplies is similar to extending the control of the purchasing department over any other area. Certain preliminary activity by the purchasing manager is necessary.

First and most important, the full support of the hospital administration must be obtained. This may be easy, but it might require some persuasion. To become well enough informed to either convince the administration of the feasibility of controlling pharmacy purchases or to begin to develop a plan to do so, the purchasing manager should study the pharmaceutical market and current purchasing practices, talking with both vendors and in-house personnel. The manager should try to get a feel for the peculiarities of the field, loyalties, and tradition in order to understand both the facts and the subjective situation to be faced. Consultation with other purchasing managers can be very useful.

Once approval to proceed has been obtained, the purchasing manager should sit down with the director of the pharmacy and openly discuss the project. This is the opportune time to assure the director that the intent is only to apply the purchasing department's specialty to that area, which will then free up time that can be used for the advancement of the pharmacy department's specialty. If the purchasing manager fails to achieve a "calming of the nerves" effect at this meeting, the meeting should be ended on a high note and discussions continued again as soon as possible.

Before formulating a workable plan for taking control of the procurement of pharmaceuticals, the purchasing manager must accumulate much information, including:

- how the hospital is presently charged for medications;
- how the hospital charges patients for medication;
- the hospital's reimbursement procedures;
- problems with current pharmacy operations;
- medication-related problems faced by physicians and nurses;
- relevant state and federal laws and regulatory requirements; and
- accreditation requirements.

CHOOSING A STRUCTURE

The next step is to decide on the structure of purchasing activity to be followed. Purchasing departments are usually structured in one of two ways:

1. Full control, and centralized: All purchasing functions and related activities are handled by the purchasing department.
2. Full control, but decentralized: The purchasing department establishes the specific policies and procedures for control of inventories and direction of the procurement activities of other major departments within the

hospital, but it does not directly process all purchases.

Most purchasing departments presently fall into category one, but as the pressure on hospitals to contain costs increases, more and more will be gravitating toward the second category, in efforts to fulfill the various cost-containment pressures and yet not increase departmental staff levels.

The expertise of the various pharmacy departmental personnel is too important to sacrifice for the growth of a purchasing function.

If purchasing can fully exercise its expertise and at the same time involve the expertise of the department being affected, it can expand its sphere of activity and control without the usual power struggles, which only serve to divide rather than unite.

If the centralized approach is chosen, the following steps must be taken.

- Develop appropriate product listings containing complete product descriptions, units of purchase, and units of issue.
- Establish a list of acceptable manufacturers for each line item or grouping.
- Learn about any particular delivery requirements or manufacturer/distributer stocking requirements.

Obviously, developing this information will require much discussion with the pharmacy director as well as with vendors.

If the decentralized approach is chosen, policies must be established on:

- when written bids are required;
- method of receipt of materiel into the hospital;
- procedure for monitoring activity;
- returned goods;

- product recalls; and
- invoice approvals.

In the following discussion it will be assumed that a "full control, but decentralized" system is in force.

The purchasing manager must then assemble adequate personnel to supervise pharmaceutical purchases and inventory control. The staff should be provided with a written procedure manual to ensure uniformity of processes and compliance with all statutes and regulations.

INVENTORY PROCEDURES

Establishing centralized control over the pharmaceutical inventory is similar to doing so for any kind of supplies. The objective of any pharmaceutical procurement and distribution system is to get the items at the lowest price, store them safely, and get them to end users on request. A list of the 25 to 50 fastest moving items should be generated and analyzed through the use of historical data obtained from other hospitals in the area, or an outside pharmaceutical organization.

At this point, the data-processing manager should be asked to help set up a computer system for handling the inventory and expected growth as it occurs. This step is essential, if a computer is available, since it will save a great deal of time in the future. If a computer is not available, a system of traveling requisitions for each item should be set up. (Traveling requisitions are permanent transaction records showing descriptions of routinely used items, acceptable vendors, previous purchase information, and pricing levels.)

It should be determined what stock levels are to be maintained for those 25 to 50 items. Usually, at first a one-month supply is more than adequate. It is important to figure in the order and delivery times needed for stock replenishment. A constant physical inventory system should be followed to determine actual usage compared to original estimates, and appropriate changes in stock levels should be made. Gradually more items can be added to the inventory, as space and experience dictate. It is extremely important that the purchasing department monitor its purchases of items, so as to be able to avail itself of the EOQ (economic order quanti-

---

A constant physical inventory system should be followed to determine actual usage compared to original estimates, and appropriate changes in stock levels should be made.

---

ty), EOV (economic order value), and/or ROP (reorder point) formulae in order to achieve the optimum, or most advantageous pricing levels for that item.

The problem of not knowing when a physician will switch from one medication to another is common to all forms of pharmaceutical purchasing. Therefore, purchasers must remain current in their knowledge of the industry and procedures in order to be able to move freely and at a moment's notice. Sudden changes in medication use may leave the pharmacy with a stock of merchandise that is no longer usable. In such a case the purchasing manager should contact the major

distributor for help in alleviating the problem. This can be done through the other customers the distributor sells to.

Bidding and contracts

A one-year guarantee on price should be sought from all bidders. Where possible, orders should be combined and a prime vendor agreement reached. It is desirable to bid items through the manufacturer, then bid through the distributor. The distributor will usually lower the price, depending on the volume of business to be done. All purchase contracts should include a "credit clause" whereby the conditions are preset for returning merchandise that is not acceptable.

One of the greatest problems will be price fluctuation. A system must be established to monitor the changes as they occur. If there is ever doubt about what a price is or whether a price is competitive, the American Druggist *Blue Book,* published annually by the Hearst Corporation, can be consulted.

VENDOR SELECTION

Vendor selection is of the utmost importance. Often the purchasing manager is tempted to question the selection of one or two vendors by the pharmacists as their major sources of pharmaceuticals, when there are literally hundreds willing to serve. The truth is that there may be hundreds willing to serve, but when properly evaluated, only a few vendors will be found to provide adequate products and service.

To protect the purchasing manager and the hospital from liability, a procedure must be established for evaluating and selecting vendors in a fair and objective manner. Thorough investigation of the product and manufacturer is fully warranted, because all manufacturers do not use the same formulations to produce a particular product, and because federal regulation does not mean that unacceptable manufacturing practices have been eradicated.

Shown in Figure 1 is a sample of the document used by Detroit Medical Center Shared Services Cooperative in evaluating vendors. All vendors are required to complete one of these forms before any

PHARMACEUTICAL MANUFACTURER'S QUALITY ASSESSMENT

I. Company information
Name and address of firm
State the names and addresses of any parent or subsidiary firm (attach copy).
Name of corporate president or representative (state title).
Include an organizational chart of the company with departmental progression.
Telephone numbers:
Purchasing:
Medical and product information:
Normal hours:
After hours (emergency):
Company representative (name, address, and telephone):
a) District manager
b) Area representative
c) Alternate area representative
d) Representative in charge of Hospital Contracts
Can your products be bought direct from the company or must they be bought from wholesaler?
If direct, where is your closest shipping point?
If wholesaler, which local wholesalers?
Do you have a catalog with all your products available? (Please send one if available.)
(If catalog is unavailable, please list your products with trade name, generic name, strength.)

Figure 1. Sample vendor information document. Source: Detroit Medical Center Shared Services Cooperative, Inc. (Reprinted with permission.)

business is transacted. This screening represents an attempt to compile information about a company and its policies, along with product history data. It provides the important information needed to make preliminary decisions, information that would not be available through the sales representative.

RECEIVING PROCEDURES

Receipt of merchandise is one of the most important materiel management functions. To ensure proper, untroubled receipt the purchasing manager must:

- notify suppliers that merchandise is to be shipped in unmarked containers, so as not to draw attention to the products in each box (for example, the Rifkin Safe System, under which the pharmacy boxes are delivered to the dock in locked condition, could be utilized);
- see that the person who does the receiving is a most trusted employee, and assign that person to the receiving of pharmaceuticals on a permanent basis (some institutions rotate their "trusted" employees on a weekly basis, as to avoid devious plans for theft);
- make certain that the receiver is a different person from the checker;
- take the necessary steps so that once goods arrive at the pharmacy, a separate person will receive the materiel into pharmacy.

Any discrepancies on an order must be noted on the company driver's delivery receipt, the purchase order, the receiving slip, and when necessary or applicable, reported to a federal agency.

Pharmacy inventory should be taken at least once per week, since theft does not wait for a holiday. Narcotics and other controlled substances must be inventoried weekly, with spot verifications being made each time an order is dispensed. Since this area is so sensitive and highly regulated, it is best to have silent alarms installed and activated during off duty hours. According to the Federal Drug Enforcement Agency, all narcotics and controlled substances must be kept under lock and key. It is also recommended that they be interspersed throughout the pharmacy stock so as to make theft more difficult. At no time is there to be a floor stock of narcotics—with the exception of cardiac and shock treatment drugs, which must be under lock and key on the floor area.

DISTRIBUTION PROCEDURES

Policies and procedures on distribution of drugs and prescriptions are very important. The following is a sample procedure to follow for ensuring safety:

1. Physician-ordered prescriptions are forwarded to the pharmacy in any convenient manner.
2. The pharmacist fills the prescriptions and delivers them to the respective floor areas.
3. The pharmacist solicits a signature from the nurse in charge, stating that he or she has received whatever was delivered.
4. Any notices of refills on medication must be accompanied by the empty bottle or container in order to be replenished.
5. All floor drugs must be kept under lock and key.

6. Drug/medication sheets should be used. These should state who gave what to whom and at what time, with what dosage left to administer.
7. A formulary committee should be established. Its main purpose is to take responsibility for the continuity of drugs and medications consistent with new medical techniques.
8. Ordering of pharmaceuticals can be done once per week, or at whatever interval is more convenient.
9. The purchasing agent must decide on which housekeeping person will clean the pharmacy and the times it will be done.

GENERIC DRUGS

The formulary committee also would be responsible for reviewing and judging the acceptance of generic drugs. It would approve the use of specific generic drugs for certain brand name drugs. The formulary committee (or therapeutics committee, in some hospitals) sets the specifications on drugs and what they will accept as substitutes, within a given range. One of the committee's main jobs, of course, is to promote the acceptance and use of generics. However, some pharmacies complain about the quality of generics—indicating a

The formulary committee would be responsible for reviewing and judging the acceptance of generic drugs. It would approve the use of specific generic drugs for certain brand name drugs.

definite need for the formulary committee.

For example, the product tetracycline has about five different manufacturers, each making slight variations in the product. By establishing the parameters of operation, the list of acceptable products can be reduced, possibly, to two or three.

FURTHER INNOVATION

Once a controlled system for purchasing, storing, and distributing pharmaceuticals has been instituted, the hospital administration can call a halt to major innovations or it may approve further measures to improve the control of drugs. Two systems in particular increase control tremendously because they return the responsibility for drug and medication safety to the pharmacy where it belongs and leave the nurses free to perform their jobs: an IV additive program, and unit-dose packaging.

Under the IV additive program, all additives to IVs are made in the pharmacy under sterile, controlled conditions. The mixtures are checked and rechecked for accuracy. The same procedures for handling drug deliveries to the floor are followed under this program. A major benefit of this type of program is that it removes the possibility of the theft of additives before they get to the patient.

The unit-dose system is the next system

to implement. Its purpose is to have the pharmacist prepare all drugs and medications, including injectables, in the pharmacy and send them up to the floor area. Only enough medication for each dose or a one day controlled supply is sent. Theft is kept to a minimum, since the system makes it almost impossible for someone to steal part of a medication, especially if the medication sheets are used.

The only loophole is the distribution of commonly used pain relief tablets (PRNs) since the quantity each patient will use cannot be predicted. However, the usual dosage is one every four hours. A separate monitoring system can be established to monitor usage by each patient by means of a special check-off sheet which can be devised by the pharmacy.

There are sources with whom a hospital can contract for help in setting up a new system. One of them is the state pharmaceutical association, which will either come into the hospital and guide management through the steps necessary to implement various systems, or suggest consultants who will undertake this task.

Establishing a pharmaceutical procurement system is not really difficult. The basic prerequisites are cooperation and communication among the parties involved and a commitment to getting the job done. The commitment level is rising in most hospitals as more and more emphasis is being placed on cost reduction or containment.

Understanding economic order quantity

Bruce G. Haywood
Vice President
Operations
Methodist Hospitals of Memphis
Memphis, Tennessee

IN ORDER to fully understand and discuss the effective use of the "quantity factor" as a tool in a controlled, organized overall inventory management system, it is essential to first understand (1) the importance of the inventory as it relates to the total financial investment of the institution as a whole and (2) the basic purpose served by inventories.

It is important that materiel managers of an extremely large asset of an institution fully recognize their responsibility and are able to control this asset to the advantage of the institution—both to ensure financial stability and to contribute to the success of its operations. Materiel managers must recognize and strive for perfect inventory balance and recognize the relationships of one inventory item to another.

Factors that can cause inventory imbalance include:

1. failure to review and revise, as necessary, inventory policies on a regular basis;

2. failure to participate in a program of long-range planning and policy determination;
3. failure of the system to react to rapid changes in usage or to accurately forecast future needs and requirements;
4. failure to develop adequate sources of supply, breakdowns in transportation, etc.;
5. failure to gain the cooperation and assistance of using departments and to properly determine their needs and direction of operation;
6. lack of standardization;
7. failure to base buying on actual needs or scientific facts;
8. failure to obtain and train appropriate personnel; and
9. inability to comprehend and to utilize the mathematical and scientific tools of inventory control such as reorder points, economic order quantity (EOQ), etc.

Others in the materiel management field could undoubtedly add to this list: All materiel managers have seen the problems associated with a poorly organized and run inventory system which results in overstock, or understock, shortages to operating departments, high procurement costs, low return on investments, etc. Thus it is essential to recognize and combat the underlying causes of inventory imbalance. Materiel managers must be cautious not to succumb to such pressures and standards, which in themselves are only meant as yardsticks. As an example, managers too often succumb to pressures to increase the inventory turnover—that is, the ratio of inventory to annual usage—to reduce inventories. While inventory turnover can be used as one of several indicators to judge the efficient use of the inventory investment, it must be simply utilized on a comparative basis with other years, institutions, etc. Turnover should always be governed by sound purchasing practices. If managers consider turnover but not safety or economy, the advantages of quantity buying and an uninterrupted supply to the using departments will be forgotten. Managers are again faced with one of the most important facets of purchasing and inventory control management: the purchase of the most economical quantity. Consequently, just as they have found that there is just the right quality item to purchase, they find that there is also exactly the right quantity to purchase.

There is a constant challenge to reduce inventories to a minimum level—not only to maintain the operating efficiency of the institution but also to anticipate delivery problems, maintain maximum discounts for merchandise, anticipate seasonal problems, account for vendor delays, etc. The importance of the total size of the inventories cannot be overstated in terms of its influence on the institution's cash flow, operating expenses and overall fiscal stability. Many industrial companies have failed because of excess inventories. It is important to remember that these invento-

The importance of the total size of the inventories cannot be overstated in terms of its influence on the institution's cash flow, operating expenses and overall fiscal stability.

ries represent not only dollar restrictions in cash flow; they also require additional capital for storage, utilities, insurance and the myriad of associated overhead expenses.

THE IMPORTANCE OF INVENTORY SIZE

It should be noted that too large an inventory ties up large amounts of cash (and quite possibly interest on that cash) which otherwise could be utilized in the operation for other purposes. It increases the chances of such negative factors as obsolescence, deterioration and damage. However, too low an inventory can create reduced efficiency in the operation, increased cost through rush demand purchases, less than economical orders, etc. It thus becomes important for an institution to determine and maintain adequate inventories to sustain the volume of work in the institution at the optimum level of effectiveness and efficiency consistent with sound fiscal management. The inventory system should be supportive of and meet the overall needs of the institution in an effective, efficient and cost-conscious manner.

One's view of inventories varies, within the hospital, based on departmental aims and direction. Thus, while the fiscal department desires the very lowest possible inventory levels to preserve and increase the institution's cash flow, the various using departments within the institution will insist upon the highest level of inventory—with sufficient safety stocks— to preserve departmental operations under all conditions regardless of cost consider-

ation. The inventory control manager or purchasing officer seeks a middle-of-the-road approach to inventory control, maintaining low inventory levels, assured safety stock, low ordering costs, justifiable carrying costs and high inventory turnover. It is known, however, that as quantities ordered decrease, carrying costs are reduced while ordering costs rise; and when quantities ordered increase, the reverse is true. Thus cost of acquisition and cost of possession are two opposing factors to take into account when considering the quantity to buy for inventory.

It is important to bear in mind that basically inventories serve two general purposes in an institution—protection and economy:

1. Sufficient materiel must be stocked to meet the ongoing needs and demands of the overall institution in an efficient and effective manner (protection); and
2. Reductions in overall operating expenses through the purchase of larger, more economical quantities must be realized (economy).

There may be other factors influencing the establishment of inventories; but basically all of them will fall into one of the above classifications. Once both the concept and the fundamental purpose of all inventories are understood, the following basic factors in establishing an inventory must be faced:

1. how much stock to purchase at one time; and
2. when it should be purchased.

One involves the order quantity factor and the other the reorder point. The proper analysis of the factors bearing on these two questions and the application of sound principles will thus lead both to an effective, efficient inventory and to its control. At this point the materiel manager's main concern will be focused on the first question—how much stock to purchase at one time. As noted above, just as there is a suitable quality for materiel, or a suitable time to purchase this materiel, there is also a suitable "most economical" ordering quantity.

There is always a "right quantity" to be purchased at any given time. However, regardless of the method used, there are two basic groups of factors that are faced in determining ordering quantities:

External Factors:
1. the time the merchandise is in transit;
2. the manufacturer's production cycle and economical production quantity;
3. market trends;
4. standardized packaging or shipping quantities;
5. quantity price variations; and
6. anticipated forward purchases.

Internal Factors:
1. handling costs;
2. storage space and facilities;
3. the possibility of deterioration;
4. the cost of insurance on goods in storage;
5. the loss of cash available for other investments and interest on inventory investments;
6. the need for additional staffing (either purchasing or inventory management);
7. the possibility of obsolescence through reduced demand by a depart-

ment, discontinuation of a system or procedure, etc.;
8. any predetermined stock turnover rates; and
9. the institution's policy of forward buying or speculative purchases.

The inventory control manager or purchasing officer, or whoever controls the inventory management decisions, must be an active participant in the institution's overall planning program in order to cope with the above factors and make the best decisions for the institution. Moreover, effective inventory management depends both upon complete cooperation by all of the user departments and evaluating the two groups of factors listed above.

THE "MIN/MAX" APPROACH

A discussion of the right quantity to purchase would not be complete without a brief summary of the "min/max" (minimum/maximum levels) approach to the "quantity factor" as an alternative and comparison to the EOQ approach to quantity determination. Basically the "min/max" approach relies on the combination of two factors: (1) the order point and (2) the total quantity to be ordered. Thus the order point is the minimum level and the combination of the order point and the total order quantity is the maximum level. The figures can be expressed in days, weeks, months—or even in dollars, though variations in the cost may hamper the efficient use of this system. A simple illustration of the formula is:

Minimum level = 2 weeks
Maximum level = 6 weeks

Supplier lead time = 1 week
Order quantity   = 4 weeks

Therefore, in order to maintain a maximum level of a six-week supply, the order must be placed when the level on hand is at three-weeks (one-week supplier lead time plus two-week minimum level); but the order must not exceed a four-week supply so that the maximum level will not be exceeded. There are advantages as well as serious disadvantages to this method:

1. It provides protection against unusual upswings because of the minimum requirement. Moreover, the minimum level may be either too low or too high for some items.

2. It ensures that there will not be excesses in stock because of the maximum level factors. It does not, however, take into consideration inventory holding costs, cost to issue a purchase order, unit cost of an item, etc.

3. It is fairly easy to monitor and understand and can be easily explained and justified. However, it does not take into consideration such things as quantity purchases for discounts and rapid changes in usage. Furthermore, it makes no use of a systematic or mathematical approach to the determination of the best order sizes.

The disadvantages of the "min/max" approach to quantity determination far outweigh the advantages. Consequently, despite its limitations, the mathematical approach to determination of the most economical order size is by far the superior method.

In determining the most economical ordering quantity many factors are taken into consideration in addition to the basic need for the item. These include factors such as those shown earlier in this article, under the two basic groups, plus unit cost of the item in various quantities, the number of purchasing orders (POs) issued and the cost per PO, inventory carrying cost, and average inventory based on different purchases. There have been a number of different formulas, all practical and workable, to mathematically determine EOQ. However, the basic concept and definition of EOQ can be said to be that order quantity which will minimize both ordering costs and inventory carrying cost. Thus this can now be translated into one of the more widely accepted formulas as a guide for further analysis and discussion. (See Figure 1.) It must be remembered that the formula is valuable only if the two cost factors can be determined with a reasonable degree of accuracy. However, many hospitals find that they do not have detailed information either on the order cost (total cost to issue a purchase order) or the inventory carrying cost. Thus, it is necessary to employ a relatively simple method to determine these two factors.

In order to ensure the viability of the EOQ formula it is essential that the determination of the two cost variables be as accurate as possible. Generally the information on inventory carrying cost is available in hospital accounting departments. Moreover, the order cost can be easily calculated by purchasing with a little bit of work plus all of the pertinent facts. To determine the inventory carrying cost it will be necessary to know, in terms of square footage of storage for each item:

1. utility costs;

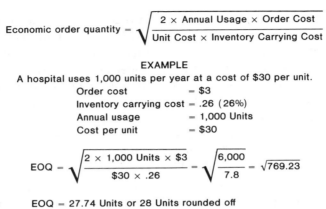

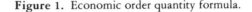

Figure 1. Economic order quantity formula.

2. maintenance cost;
3. building depreciation;
4. shelving and bin storage cost; and
5. cleaning cost.

The total cost per square foot of storage is multiplied by the total number of square feet. Then, to arrive at the storage cost as a percent of inventory, this total storage cost is divided by the current average inventory value. Finally, the other holding costs are totaled as a percentage of inventory value such as insurance, loss through obsolescence, deterioration, theft, etc., and cost of capital (how much could be made on the money if there was no inventory at all).

EXAMPLE:

Insurance	1%
Obsolescence, deterioration, theft	1%
Cost of capital	8%
Storage cost	16%
Total holding cost percentage	26%

Now to go back to the original EOQ example:

Per square foot cost total	= $2.50
Total square feet of storage	= 20,000
Current inventory value	= $300,000

Cost as a percent of inventory	= 16%
Additional holding cost factors	= 10%
Total holding cost percent	= 26%

Much of the raw data cited above can be obtained from the hospital's fiscal department and then assembled and calculated by the inventory control manager or purchasing officer. It might be noted that all stock will not necessarily have the same carrying cost. Items such as perishable foods and certain pharmaceuticals will generally have higher carrying or holding costs because of special storage facilities, additional security restrictions, additional utilities, etc., than items such as forms and office supplies. Thus the materiel manager may want to determine carrying or holding costs on several classifications of inventory and not utilize a single percentage figure.

THE ORDER COST FORMULA

Determining the ordering cost can be quite simple unless an extensive cost analysis is desired. In the absence of such an extensive cost analysis (1) take all of the yearly salaries and expenses in purchasing, (2) add in all of the accounts payable expenses directly attributable to processing invoices for payment and (3) divide by the total number of purchase orders issued per year. Then divide by the average number of items per order to determine the cost per line item. Returning to the EOQ example discussed above:

Total expense of purchasing plus accounts payable (invoice processing portion only) per year = $96,000

Total number of purchase orders issued per year = 8,000

Average cost per purchase order = $ 12

Average number of line items per purchase order = 4

Average order cost per line item = $ 3

The necessary figures can be easily obtained from purchasing or from the hospital's fiscal department. It is important to remember when determining wages to include all pertinent fringe benefits and when determining other expenses to include any allocations for lights, heat, telephone, etc., in the calculations.

When the EOQ on any individual line item has been determined, it should rarely change unless the variables change. Furthermore, after working with the mathematical formula the materiel manager may wish to set up a table, graph or chart based on the constant values of the inventory carrying cost and the order cost, thus greatly simplifying the procedure and speeding up the calculation determination.

Once materiel managers have all the variables associated with determining EOQ and understand the advantages and limitations, etc., they are ready to use the formula effectively in their own institutions. They have applied the principles of EOQ, taking into consideration all of the other quantity factors discussed earlier (e.g., price fluctuations based on quantity discounts, storage limitations, obsolescence). Once the EOQ principle has been applied, managers will quickly see the effect on their institutions of a perfectly balanced inventory that is (1) very simple

---

Once the EOQ principle has been applied, managers will quickly see the effect on their institutions of a perfectly balanced inventory.

---

and easy to explain; (2) flexible (it can be altered as conditions dictate); (3) accurate (it is based on mathematical, scientific information, not on instinct or judgment) and (4) timely (it reacts to the needs of the institution). It also has a good stock turnover (keeping shortages to a minimum and eliminating obsolete and deteriorated inventories). At this point, materiel managers will be able to scientifically and mathematically justify their inventory systems and their inventory levels.

Understanding the principles of supply consignment

Kathryn C. Maurer
Buyer, Medical-Surgical Supplies
Saint Francis Hospital
Tulsa, Oklahoma

TO BUY or not to buy? This question is sometimes easily answered in day-to-day life; but in the area of health care, it becomes infinitely more difficult. This is in part due to the fact that materiel managers must make decisions about what to buy, how much to buy and when to buy.

WHAT IS THE SUPPLY CONSIGNMENT PRINCIPLE?

In the context in which it is used in this article, the verb "to consign" means to hand over, to give, transfer or deliver formally. The supply consignment principle used in hospital inventory can be defined as those goods or services maintained in inventory stock at no cost until expressly used, at which time payment comes due. Consigned supplies may be located both in various departments and in many facets of goods and services. Outside of the hospital setting, consignments occur in everyday marketing. A jeweler, for example, receives many precious items on consignment and pays upon sale of each consigned good. In other words, it is not until the jeweler sells the merchandise to the consumer that a sale from vendor to dealer is consummated. In the hospital, the materiel manager consummates the commitment to pay only when such goods or service have been "sold" to the patient. Maintenance of inventory in the materiel manager's hands assures access to the goods wherever necessary. Title, however, remains with the vendor until needed and passed to the end user. In order to promote the principle of supply consignment, the entire stock of inventories throughout the institution must be independently evaluated.

WHERE CAN THE CONSIGNMENT METHOD BE USED?

A variety of items is purchased and consumed within the materiel environment daily. Low volume–high dollar, high volume–low dollar, high volume–high dollar, and low volume–low dollar items comprise a menagerie to evaluate. In a survey of midwestern facilities, the author found several items to be consistently promoted for consignment supply (see Table 1). High dollar–low volume items were almost unanimously promoted under the consignment procedures. This category is exemplified primarily by pacemakers, leads, transmitters and similar items. An item that has diminished in actual promotion was found to be the orthopedic prosthesis components. The trend appears to be away from consignment supply because companies are tightening the rein on their products. Although the Medical Device Amendments of 1976 (PL 94-295) has been cited for the decline, this appears to be the decoy for limiting consigned stock.

Another example of rental consignment found in the survey is the consigned use of transcutaneous nerve stimulators. Here, the units are furnished by dealers at no charge to promote their products. After becoming acquainted with the unit, patients elect their brand preference and are then permitted to take the unit home when discharged. In this situation, purchase billing is between patient and company. (Hospitals may indicate a local dealer from whom the unit may be purchased. In this concept, hospital units are consigned from the dealer for product familiarity and introduction to the patient.)

A new aspect of marketing medical-surgical expendables has recently been developed. One national dealer is selling a consignment program under the auspices of good materiel management. The high-volume, expendable medical-surgical supplies are relatively new to the consignment principle in comparison with the other categories. Represented are primarily the fast-turn, lower dollar type items. But a word of caution: There appears a need to be more cautious in this area than in any other evaluated.

Another aspect of disposable medical-surgical supplies is one used at Saint Francis Hospital in Tulsa, Oklahoma. (See Table 1.) Disposable operating room (OR) packs and gowns are on a bid-type consignment program. All necessary products are brought into stores without billing

Table 1. Middle west survey of products received on consignment

Name of Facility	Zimmer Prosthesis	Medline Medical Products	Stryker Pads	Converters Packs and Gowns	Medtronics Pacemakers	Intramedics Pacemakers	Telectronic Pacemakers	Precision Cosmet Lens	DePuy Prosthesis	Trans Nerve Stimulators	Scientific Products (lab equipment)	Cardiac Pacemaker	Arco Pacemakers	Cordis Pacemakers	Medcor Pacemakers
Oklahoma Osteopathic Tulsa, Okla.	XX				XX				XX						
Saint Francis Hospital Tulsa, Okla.			XX	XX	XX		XX			XX	XX				
Doctor's Hospital Tulsa, Okla.		XX													
Washington Regional Fayetteville, Ark.					XX					XX					
Rogers Memorial Rogers, Ark.					XX	XX									
Baptist Medical Oklahoma City, Okla.					XX	XX	XX						XX	XX	XX
Saint John's Hospital Joplin, Mo.	XX							XX	XX						
L.E. Cox Medical Springfield, Mo.					XX										

and are not billed until the number of surgical and obstetrical cases in a month's period has been tabulated. Thereafter, billing is calculated per procedure—surgical and obstetrical—for a total month's billing. Cost per procedure is bid firm for each one-year term of a two-year contract.

Purchase by use is the method of paying for how much a piece of equipment or asset is used. (For example, a copier may be rated by the number of copies made during a month's period.) Use of this technique reduces costs for equipment that is not in continual use for which outright purchase is infeasible, by limiting payment to the actual use of equipment.[1]

Before consignment as a principle can be evaluated, advantages and disadvantages must be examined. Advantages lie in favor of the materiel manager and oftentimes the vendor, as in the following situations:

1. on new types of goods when the acceptance cannot be adequately estimated;
2. for low-volume items; and
3. where quantities are uncertain and shortlived.[2]

After examining the advantages of the new system of consigned products, the following potential disadvantages inherent in this form of purchase should be scrutinized.

THE POTENTIAL ADVANTAGES AND PITFALLS OF UTILIZING CONSIGNED ITEMS

1. Immediate dollar savings can be easily identified by a 30-day accounts payable lag. It is essential to work for the best possible price. Like commitments of guaranteed prices for the institutional term period are a must. Price increases should be scrutinized carefully to protect the integrity of any new system. Savings must be actual net—not gross.

2. Consignment programs should be considered on the basis of the overall effect they will have on the internal operations of the hospital. Marketed labor-saving, paper-flow programs should be

---

Consignment programs should be considered on the basis of the overall effect they will have on the internal operations of the hospital.

---

analyzed for possible overstocking situations and actual warehousing of the vendor's product. Total overhead costs, including costs of inventory control of materiel warehousing, are necessary in an honest presentation of savings. The materiel manager must guard against a laxity of vendor control. Blanket orders and stockouts are possible, regardless of whether or not a system of consignment is used. Alternate sources should be available on all possible commodity items, notwithstanding any consignment program. Freight is detrimental to overall account-

ability. Unless special handling or extraordinary circumstances arise, all goods should be bid or obtained "FOB: Destination." The firm is then responsible for all claims, damages, shortages, etc. A fair comparison of bids is possible whenever freight is included in the net price. In this way, if shopping or bidding, the materiel manager causes freight to be a negotiable rather than an inflexible factor. The most conjective vendor is then negotiating the hospital's freight factor in addition to competing on manufacturer's price.

3. Each department must determine an adequate safety stock and move toward minimum stocks in a prudent buyer-type program. If marketed consignment appears stock heavy on the proposed 30-day basis using department must align levels toward a minimum safety with a workable reorder period. If five-day safety is necessary due to internal control, order quantities, order points, etc., these things must be considered when determining proper economic order quantities and order points. A danger in consignment stock buying is that buyers may stock their shelves with what might be less than desirable merchandise.[3] One should counter a consignment program proposal to the vendor with turn of stock on a weekly basis or bimonthly turn.

Use of consignment was customary in several services in the midwestern hospitals which were surveyed. Services were provided at no charge until the end of the month. Billing was contingent upon quantities used. For example, laboratory equipment was furnished at no charge, with billing at end of month (EOM) of actual tests run for a fixed charge per tests for reagents. Reagents are thus consigned until tests are counted at the period's end and then become due. Another service common to consignment is a particular flotation pad on the market. Rental is not predetermined; rather, it is dependent upon actual patient days utilized. Billing is made at EOM after the number of patient days is tallied per identified flotation pad. Once again, revenue is billed before actual payable comes due.

As these three areas of supplies under consignment are examined they appear to be a very adaptable purchasing technique throughout the institution. Several precautions should, however, be stressed: From individual patient items to entire product categories, to and including equipment, provisions must be made for continuity in the definition of consignment.

ENTERING THE WORLD OF CONSIGNMENT

The consignment process is very easy to begin once the administration, the materiel manager and the using department determine that it is beneficial to and desirable for their institution. The category or items to be consigned should be selected. The quantities needed of each particular item by the end user should be enumerated. Once quantities are calculated, considering lead times and usage, the vendor(s) must be solicited. The negotiating expertise of the materiel manager becomes evident. The success of the ensuing negotiations is dependent upon the commitment to the consignment principle. Once one single vendor of a multiple within the category

responds with a positive proposal, the puzzle will fall into place. Needless to say, not one vendor will want competitors to offer a proposal as easy as consignment and not be able to respond. Caution in exercising unfulfilling ploys should be guarded against. Only bona fide requests should be made in all circumstances. Those items that are high dollar–low volume will probably gain the fastest support from administration, department and vendor. Ironically, the smaller hospital may have an unknown advantage since in reality only a small amount of inventory may be needed at any one time. Record keeping might be less complex in the smaller institution where smaller consignment quantities are maintained.

To undertake the consignment principle, one of the following methods should be selected: (1) attrition-out the already-purchased stock and bring in new consigned stock for replacement or (2) have the vendor purchase back all product on-hand-inventory and issue credit for the dollar amount to be consigned.

Of the three methods discussed above, the second option appears to be the hardest to negotiate. It is, however, perhaps the most effective way to start. Vendors may overreact to their company entering this "losing" market style and having to give credit; but in the long run, the advantages of the system should more than prevail for both parties.

The consignment principle may be somewhat underused in the sales field, but this need not be the case. Personnel in materiel management should evaluate the principle in every imaginative situation within their jurisdiction and test the market. They should investigate the various options in the marketplace and pursue them.

Consignment purchasing ... one potentially workable answer to negotiable voluntary efforts available to each and every materiel manager.

REFERENCES

1. Higgins, L. R. *Cost Reduction from A to Z* (New York: McGraw-Hill 1976) p.342.

2. Diamond, J. *Retail Buying* (Englewood Cliffs, N.J.: Prentice-Hall 1976) p.201.

3. Ibid.

Vendors: a product inservice goldmine

Edward L. Bosak, Jr.
Midwest Area Sales Manager
American V. Mueller Division
American Hospital Supply Corporation
Niles, Illinois

IN TODAY'S marketplace with its extreme cost containment sensitivity, it is important that those areas wherein expenses and basic costs of operations can be cut are identified. All too often the potentials that exist for increasing productivity are overlooked. One of the most obvious opportunities in this area comes from viewing product vendors as an "inservice goldmine."

Materiel managers must question whether they are taking full advantage of their vendor relationships. This question often precipitates an automatic affirmative answer. However, a critical look at the service capabilities of vendors vs. customers' utilization of those capabilities would reveal, in most cases, some very distinct possibilities for using vendor resources more effectively.

VENDOR RESOURCES

Technical Resources

Each vendor should be viewed by the institution as a technical resource. As a supplier of a product or a service, a vendor will maintain information on a specific product or group of products. This information may include specifications, clinical studies, instructions for use, and instructions for care and maintenance. In a highly technical market such as the health care industry, it is difficult if not impossible for everyone to keep up with technical advancements, but vendors can be an important source of information.

Human Resources

Vendors also offer human resources. Vendors often have highly trained individuals available to conduct inservice training on specific products. It is not unusual for vendor representatives to assist in portions of nursing school curricula. Subjects such as the care and handling of surgical instruments or the care and maintenance of the surgical microscope are examples of product inservices that are valuable in nursing education. In addition, technically experienced individuals such as operating room nurses, anesthesiologists, or surgeons may be retained by the vendor as consultants, and the expertise of these individuals is available to materiel managers.

Supportive Resources

Vendors should be viewed as support organizations. Vendors will quite often be able to supply technical films, books, articles, etc. to be used as resource material, training material, or as in the case of a surgical case cart system, guidelines for the development of an individual specialized system.

THE VENDOR'S POINT OF VIEW

Many vendors view product inservice as an opportunity to contact people who are not seen on a regular basis. Primary customers for V. Mueller are operating room personnel; representatives normally have the opportunity to talk with the operating room supervisor or selected members of the staff. Other than product inservice, there are few opportunities to speak with the general operating room staff. Through these inservices, the company is able to demonstrate its ability to solve problems and answer questions. Some call this "goodwill" but it is also common sense.

Getting the Message Across

The rapport that is developed between the company representative and the hospital staff is a definite plus in the eyes of a vendor. There is an old saying, "A fact is only a fact if your listener believes you." Although the company conveys its message through literature, personal letters, and similar means, there is nothing like a face-to-face meeting to ensure that the message is being received. Product inservice is an excellent vehicle for the achievement of this end.

Gaining a Competitive Advantage

Quite often, product inservice performed in the past confers a "competitive advantage." In many cases, given identical or very comparable pricing, the past record of service and the willingness to work with the customer is enough to tilt the balance. So, it rapidly becomes obvious that there are positive benefits of product inservice for both the vendor and the customer.

Improving Productivity

There are several areas in which vendors and hospitals can improve productivity through the use of product inservice. The first of these is "need recognition." It is virtually impossible to develop a product or a service until the function of that product or service has been defined. An excellent example of this is the Operating Room Utilization Program recently intro-

---

The introduction of a new product will normally create a need for product inservice, and it is the responsibility of the vendor to ensure that inservice training is available.

---

duced by V. Mueller. The need delineated in this program was twofold: (1) to control more effectively surgical instrument inventory and (2) to control more effectively time and facility utilization in the operating room.

Once these needs were defined, the development of the program to satisfy them could progress. Similarly, the introduction of a new product will normally create a need for product inservice, and it is the responsibility of the vendor to ensure that inservice training is available. There are hundreds of products that would be useless to the institution were it not for the training and information provided by the vendor.

Program production is a major expense and effort on the part of the vendor. Hundreds of thousands of dollars are spent annually by vendors in the production of product inservice programs. For example, a 12-minute film demonstrating the use of a new surgical instrument or the care and handling of that instrument can easily cost more than $50,000. The logistics involved in the production of such a film can be staggering, yet these things must be accomplished to market and service the product effectively.

PRODUCT INSERVICE TYPES

The types of product inservice available are varied, but generally can be placed in one of the following three categories.

1. Use/function is the type of inservice that explains to the hospital staff what the function of the product is and how it is used. In most cases, there is a primary function and a secondary function. For example, a stone basket primarily designed for urology may also have application in biliary tract surgery. It is not uncommon for a customer to be unaware of a secondary function. This, of course, limits the amount of use and potential productivity derived from the product.

2. Implementation inservice may be linked with the use/function type or may be done separately. This refers to guidelines on the logical implementation of utilization of the product. An example of this is the purchase of surgical case carts. The function of the case cart may or may not be obvious both on the primary and

secondary levels. However, the implementation of the case cart as a system quite often is subject to many variances. The experience of the vendor in setting up case cart systems will prove invaluable in the implementation of the system.

3. Care and handling inservice becomes more and more complex as the technology in the health care industry increases. Hospitals invest millions of dollars annually in product and capital equipment. The maintenance of that equipment is a primary target for cost containment. The vendor should play a key role in assuring proper care and maintenance for the dollars so invested.

CUSTOMER EXPECTATIONS

First and foremost, customers should expect vendors to be an information source regarding the products and services that are purchased. In selecting vendors it is important to ensure that the information and services required will be available.

Second, updates on existing products and periodic orientation for new employees should be a part of vendors' services. Finally, vendors should be a source of guidance and innovation in the area of inservice programs. The old adage "All that glitters is not gold" is too often true. However, fully utilizing vendor product inservice capabilities can prove to be a real goldmine for customers' institutions.

Utilizing suppliers to the hospital's best interests

William K. Henning
Director of Management Consulting
American Hospital Supply Division
McGaw Park, Illinois

TWO WELL-KNOWN TYPES of hospital purchasing agents are becoming an endangered species in the cost containment environment. The compulsive bidder, who expects nothing more than "price" from vendors, is joining the "you'll get your order after you take me to lunch" purchasing agent on the road to extinction.

Both types are changing their ways or leaving the field because their old practices do not utilize vendors' capabilities to hold down the hospital's internal costs of ordering, storing and handling. Some are joining the majority of hospital purchasing agents who are doing a better job investigating the capabilities of vendors, specifying hospital service requirements to vendors, establishing simple hospital vendor ordering systems, negotiating and contracting for these services and monitoring performance to see their hospitals receive the prices and service levels in the agreement.

The old purchasing practices that

focused on product price and superficially managed vendor service resulted in higher inventories both centrally and throughout the hospital as users squirreled away products in their departments against unreliable delivery and stockouts. The higher inventories, the more purchase orders, the more back orders, and the more stockouts resulted in a supply system that could not be controlled for reliability and cost effectiveness. In the past few years, the prevailing purchase philosophy has become the consideration of *all* costs in the purchase decision: the product price, the vendor service and related hospital costs, the handling and use costs of the product itself. This has been described as the "total cost" approach to purchasing.

Section 2102 of the *Provider Reimbursement Manual,* guideline for Medicare reimbursement published by HEW, reflects this approach in its wording, which says, in part: "If the total cost, or components of total cost ... exceed what a prudent and cost-conscious buyer would incur, the excess is considered unreasonable cost...." "Reasonable cost ... takes into account both direct and indirect costs ... including normal standby costs."

HOSPITAL GOALS

Beyond competitive pricing, hospitals should demand of their suppliers reliability, service to keep hospital costs low and assistance in accomplishing the following goals:
1. competitive prices;
2. low ordering, storing, receiving and distributing costs;

3. vendor deliveries as promised over 90 percent of the time;
4. ample vendor inventory not far away;
5. reliable inbound transportation;
6. vendor accuracy in products, deliveries and paperwork;
7. vendor systems that simplify the order entry and the paperwork system and offer periodic reports for hospital purchasing and inventory management;
8. personal assistance from vendors to set up and operate the system;
9. broad product lines from vendors permitting multilines purchase orders, receivings and invoices;
10. standardization on quality, cost-effective products;
11. complete, up-to-date product information;
12. minimum amount of handling problems, returns and credits;
13. adherence to codes and regulations;
14. up-to-date information on materiel management systems and procedures.

THE SUPPLY CYCLE

To fully utilize vendors, hospital purchasing agents need to "think systems." Figure 1 shows the hospital cycle

---

To fully utilize vendors, hospital purchasing agents need to "think systems."

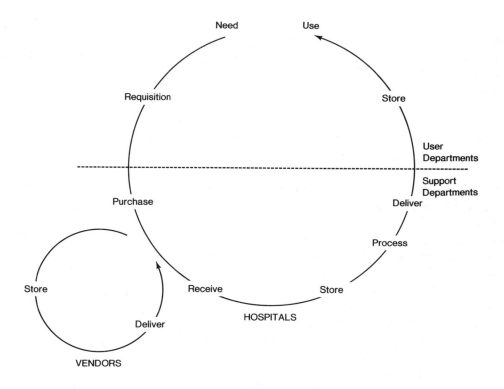

Figure 1. The supply cycle.

and its vendor's cycle joined together. Each is dependent on the other. The overall performance of the supply cycle is just as efficient as its least efficient function—vendor and hospital included.

The illustration of the hospital-vendor supply cycle shows a dotted line above which are the ordering and storing functions of the "user" departments throughout the hospital. Below the dotted line in the hospital cycle are the central purchasing, storing, receiving, processing and delivery functions of the support departments in the hospital. This illustration shows both vendor and hospital have central storage functions that for many items are a duplication of storage function.

Many purchasing agents are writing systems contracts or prime vendor agreements that permit the hospital to utilize the vendor's central storage function and reduce or eliminate the hospital's central storage function for those items.

In the old days, vendors were not considered a part of the hospital's system. Hospitals did not commit their purchases of specific products to specific vendors for periods of time so vendors had difficulty forecasting demand and building adequate inventories. As purchasing methods have included a consideration of systems, computers have assisted vendors and hospitals in assembling the product and usage information necessary to pull the hospital-vendor supply system together. With commitment and efficient systems, it is now possible for hospitals to affect their internal purchasing, holding and distributing costs dramatically.

HOSPITAL COSTS AFFECTED BY VENDOR SERVICES

We know that the average hospital spends approximately $60,000 annually to operate a single hospital bed. Of this, approximately $10,000 is spent for product and another $10,000 per bed is expended to acquire, store and distribute supplies. By his or her buying decisions, the purchasing agent affects both $10,000 per bed figures. Over the years, the average hospital has managed its procurement function to the point of having negotiated very favorable prices. Accordingly, there may be fewer cost reductions available in the $10,000 per bed product cost and far more opportunities for cost savings in the other $10,000. It follows that the available claims by hospitals of cost savings through vendor relationships describe dramatic reductions in inventory, holding costs and other operating costs.

A national distributor that has the capacity of selling $2,500 of the $10,000 per bed purchased products recently estimated that, if it were to sell the hospital all that it could at cost, this hospital would be able to reduce the cost of operating a single bed only 0.8 percent.

In addition to product prices, vendors directly affect hospital central inventories and operating costs in purchasing, receiving, general stores and accounts payable by reliable, accurate service. Indirectly, they can affect the size of "user" inventories by reliable service. Patient revenue from charge products increased by selling and helping implement exchange cart systems and product charging systems.

VENDOR-RELATED COST REDUCTION EXAMPLE

Lancaster-Fairfield County Hospital (169 beds), Lancaster, Ohio:

> Since working with "X" vendor on their prime vendor/materials management program, we have realized the following: medical, surgical and linen inventories have been reduced from $170,000 to $36,000. Including a 25 percent holding cost reduction of $33,500, this has meant a return to cash flow of $167,500.
>
> The implementation of a 24-hour cart exchange distribution program has taken lost patient charges from over $2,000 per month down to less than $300 per month.
>
> At least $14,000 annually is being saved in labor costs. At $18 per purchase order, approximately $7,200 is being saved annually in paper costs.
>
> Significant savings have also been realized in receiving and accounts payable.
>
> All of this has been realized over a two-year period while expanding from 100 to 227 beds and adding three new services.
>
> John Reid
> Administrator
> March 1978[1]

The above example of cost reduction was chosen because it illustrates the variety of costs and revenue dollars affected by a vendor-hospital relationship. It should be noted that the results were achieved through a relatively extensive relationship between vendor and hospital including several hundred products over a period of time. Purchasing agents may elect to achieve the same results by making smaller agreements with several vendors or through periodic bidding among qualified vendors. This has the effect of segmenting the system, tending to increase costs, and makes it almost impossible to calculate buying cost savings. As a result, the best "proofs of cost reduction" of hospital-vendor relationships are the ones resulting from extensive systems contracts/prime vendor agreements.

Vendors certainly can affect hospital costs negatively as well. We all know hospitals that have unconsciously built their central inventories because of poor vendor service and possibly inadequate hospital inventory management. If a hospital has its combined general stores and central supply inventories in excess of $500 per bed and less than six turns per year, it should look to its inventory management methods and its vendors' performance.

Another negative effect vendors can have is back orders. By far the worst ones are back orders not received until days or weeks after the safety factor has run out and the hospital's stock is exhausted. It has been estimated that this kind of late back order costs the hospital again as much as it originally spent to place the purchase order and process the first delivery and invoice. Depending on how automated or manual the paperwork system is, the purchase order cycle can cost from $15 to $35 per order. A late back order, because it is all manual, probably costs at least $35 to handle and incurs all kinds of stockpiling and distrust in the user departments.

GETTING THE MOST OUT OF VENDORS

Fully utilizing vendor's capabilities in the hospital's best interest requires a significant amount of study and analysis that many purchasing agents do not find time for. It is a Catch-22 situation. The agents desperately need improved systems to have time for purchasing and negotiating, yet because they have a high-transaction, manual, complex purchasing system, they don't have the time. Make the time. It will be the difference between a career as a first-class purchasing agent or materiel manager and a buyer.

The purchasing agent may have vague feelings of reluctance because he or she is unwilling or afraid to pit the power of the

Cast these feelings of reluctance and fear aside because they are costing the hospital money every day of every year.

hospital purchasing agent against the strength of certain vendors. The purchasing agent may be afraid that giving too much business to one vendor will reduce the prerogative to spread the business or offend some other vendor. Cast these feelings aside because they are costing the hospital money every day of every year. Decide to take the lead. Do enough front-end work to set up specifications that vendors must respond to. In this way, the purchasing agent states the case at first and maintains negotiating strength so satisfactory agreements for both parties result. Eventually, the hospital is working closely with its vendor to improve the efficiency of the resulting hospital/vendor system. The process is as follows:

1. Select one supplier category to investigate.

The most systems action is in the medical/surgical and laboratory areas, but you may want to start with your office suppliers or forms manufacturers.

2. Know your major vendors.

a. What is their track record? Manually or by computer periodically analyze major vendors' delivery performance to separate fact from claims and loose talk. The best approach is to have a computer inventory program that provides vendor analysis such as the display in Table 1.

b. Without computer, your office must perform manual vendor performance ratings by tabulating for each vendor:

- the total number of purchase orders in one month;
- number complete in one shipment/percent complete;
- number completed by date needed;
- average number of items per purchase order;
- number of purchase orders completed within lead time plus safety factor (usually 7–14 days);
- a rating for the period and comparison of vendors in the same product lines;
- evaluation as to whether the vendor sales representative is valuable, efficient, organized, businesslike; whether he or she knows the products, the vendor's own system and materiel management in general; whether he or she is helpful in solving problems and returning goods; whether he or she works with hospitals to reduce handling costs and standardized products.

c. Visit each major vendor.

- Check its location in regard to the hospital.
- Meet the boss and customer service representative.
- How many lines or products are offered and held in stock?
- What is the total dollar value of this inventory?
- Can it reserve stock for your hospital under a systems contract?

Table 1. Computer analysis of vendor service levels

Vendor Code	Vendor Name	Number of Receivings	Number of 100% Receivings	Total Lines Received	Lines 100% Received	Service Level
104	Kendall	1	0	25	24	96%
105	J & J	2	1	26	18	69%

- Is the warehouse orderly and clean?
- What is its trucking program?
- Does it have computer capabilities and up-to-date systems?
- Does it offer private-label products as well as national line products?
- Is is aware of the latest products, codes and regulations?

3. Investigate each vendor's system capabilities.

a. **Ordering.** For simple product lines, a simple telephone ordering service with standard product ordering numbers and standard forms is effective for small orders and few products. More and more vendors are now recommending that the hospital lease electronic transmission systems, some with card readers, to automatically and accurately transmit orders to vendors. A leading drug distributor is promoting a bar code system that permits the ordering of drugs by simply wanding the bar codes in hospital inventory.

b. **Computer System.** The ordering systems above are being eclipsed rapidly by computer input-output units in the hospital purchasing office that access vendors' computers directly. This is a major breakthrough and the beginning of significant developments in the tying together of hospital and vendor systems. Now, hospitals can place orders directly with vendor computers and receive a printed reply in the form of their own purchase order that indicates which products in the original order were back-ordered. This not only simplifies ordering

and handles the typing of the purchase order, but also indicates, particularly for outlying hospitals, which products will not be received immediately.

c. **Reports.** Vendors with computers usually provide purchasing and inventory management reports periodically that should be valuable, particularly to hospitals without their own computer capabilities. These reports show monthly usage, update reorder points (ROPs) and economic order points (EOQs) and enable the hospital purchasing agent to perform an ABC analysis of central inventory (see Appendix).

d. **Transportation.** The hospital should examine the vendor's routine schedules for delivery and the possibility of varying the schedule according to the hospital's needs.

e. **Personal Assistance.** Investigate the vendor's ability to provide personnel to help the hospital implement its new ordering system and possibly to reorganize its central storage area.

4. Define the system and estimate its cost impact on the hospital.

For the one or two vendors that look the best, describe the system on paper and try to estimate the differences in cost and performance between your present operation and using the new system. In this way specifications are developed for the negotiating sessions with the vendor. This is the process of prudent buying that evaluates the total cost effect of several alternatives.

This process will lead to the selection of

the best one or two systems and the development of specific performance goals for vendor and hospital.

5. Purchasing methods.

The purchasing agent may decide after investigation that it is not necessary for him or her to enter into a large systems contract. Possibly a blanket order will do just as well. He or she may decide to bid some items and contract for others according to which items are most price sensitive and which items benefit most from being handled in a low-cost hospital/vendor system.

It is at this time the purchasing agent should request formal proposals from vendors. Each proposal should be studied carefully and its effect on hospital operational costs examined. If these proposals are vague on service levels and other measures of performance, it is probably because the purchasing agent did not require a specific response. It is important that vendors spell out specifically what they plan to do in the area of service.

6. Monitor vendor performance.

It is hoped the purchasing agent will have initiated a format for vendor analysis in the initial phases of the search for a vendor system partner. It is then a matter of continuing to measure vendor performance to ensure that the service conditions that everyone agreed to are continued. The beginning of a vendor/hospital system relationship is probably like a new marriage. There will be bad times and happy times, but the important thing is to stick together and work out problems together.

7. Every year or two, repeat the process.

Changes in cost, vendor performance and computer systems occur continually. Prudent buying requires that the purchasing agent look over the field from time to time, and in a cost-conscious way, take a fresh look at each hospital/vendor relationship.

On the basis of the proper arm's-length negotiation for prices, products and

---

It is truly a case of 1 + 1 = 3 when hospitals and vendors get together to set up a really cost-effective supply system.

---

vendor, it is truly a case of $1 + 1 = 3$ when hospital and vendor get together to set up a really cost-effective supply system. Both hospital and vendor are committed to cost containment on a voluntary basis. As such, both are compelled to make sure the voluntary effort is successful. Within a purchasing arrangement that commits hospital and vendor, there are mutual incentives to achieve cost effectiveness and productivity toward total cost reduction.

REFERENCE

1. Communication with John Reid, Administrator, Lancaster-Fairfield County Hospital, Lancaster, Ohio, March 1978.

AMERICAN HOSPITAL SUPPLY CORPORATION

ASAP-AMERICAN
CUSTOMER USAGE REPORT

CUST. NO. 43-200-3718-005
REGION 56 SALESMAN 44
PERIOD ENDING 11/30/79
PAGE 1

CATALOG NUMBER	DESCRIPTION	ORDER QTY	UNIT OF MEAS	UNIT PRICE	LAST MONTH (NOV)	2 MOS AGO (OCT)	3 MOS AGO (SEP)	4 MOS AGO (AUG)	5 MOS AGO (JUL)	6 MOS AGO (JUN)	7 MOS AGO (MAY)	8 MOS AGO (APR)	9 MOS AGO (MAR)	10 MOS AGO (FEB)	11 MOS AGO (JAN)	12 MOS AGO (DEC)	LAST 4 MOS AVG UNITS	LAST 4 MOS AVG $	EOQ	RQP
46870-110	SHLD GOWN PACK 510 1EA/PK LGE	20	CS	46.70	95	85	80	80	83	140	80	80	115	100	110	75	85	3969	13	35
30000-100	S/O/P BASIC PACK 100 STERILE	8	CS	51.45	40	40	40	40	41	41	16	16	25	58	36	36	38	1955	38	19
65375-200	ADULT ECG MONITORING BACKPAD	6	BX	99.50	18	18	12	18	8	16	16	16	25	0	0	0	17	1641	4	10
30066-010	S/O/P SHEETS 57X80 8349 STRL	8	CS	35.28	40	40	35	35	32	32	32	36	48	36	29	29	37	1296	10	18
46979-010	SHLD ISOL GOWN 3152 N-STRL	14	CS	32.55	68	28	14	42	31	12	36	36	47	24	12	0	38	1236	11	19
30005-560	S/O/P LAPAROTOMY PACK 135 STR	8	CS	77.56	16	3	16	24	21	16	16	16	28	18	12	12	15	1144	4	10
65418-005	NDM ELECTSURG GROUNDING PAD	24	BX	19.00	72	48	48	72	48	48	48	48	72	18	72	21	60	1140	18	27
23008-020	4C INST TRAY-SHARP/BLUNT SCIS	8	CS	59.00	16	16	16	24	32	18	18	18	18	12	19	6	18	1062	6	11
47730-030	AMER SHOE COVER W/O COND STRI	8	CS	40.22	27	21	16	32	32	20	20	16	16	20	20	24	24	965	8	13
65376-010	SILVON ECG ELECTRODE-1EA/PK	30	BX	16.50	60	60	60	90	90	90	65	30	0	20	0	24	68	933	20	29
30046-415	S/O/P LIMB SHEET 8415 STERILE	4	CS	49.07	8	16	12	16	8	12	12	16	16	8	12	6	13	637	5	9
30058-540	S/O/P SPLIT SHEET 8431 STERIL	5	CS	41.72	10	10	15	15	12	15	15	20	20	5	13	13	15	625	6	10
46870-140	SHLD GOWN PACK 540 1EA/PK XLG	10	CS	49.13	10	10	10	10	10	20	20	10	23	0	10	10	13	614	6	10
43159-070	AMER HI-LO ENDO TB 7.0MM,28FR	10	BX	24.56	20	20	30	30	20	30	23	27	30	20	25	0	25	614	10	14
42480-075	STERI-STRIP SKIN CLOSURE-1/2X	8	BX	37.25	16	8	16	24	15	16	0	16	16	16	16	0	16	595	7	10
SPR54278	S56 EPIDURAL TRAY-LOS HOSP.	12	CS	96.70	8	0	8	8	0	8	0	0	0	0	0	0	6	580	2	7
22815-530	PH EXAM GLOVES-100/DISP 8X ME	60	BX	4.84	130	60	60	120	120	120	120	120	120	180	60	0	105	508	47	42
842901	URINE COLLECTOR	5	CS	60.00	5	10	10	5	10	10	0	0	10	0	0	0	8	457	4	7
30060-422	S/O/P THYROID SHEET 8422 STRL	2	CS	50.02	12	7	4	13	3	12	10	8	10	10	4	2	9	450	4	7
43717-025	LGE BOUF CAP,75EA/DISP BX,BLU	2	CS	72.54	10	4	4	6	4	4	2	2	6	6	4	2	18	435	3	11
43159-080	AMER HI-LO ENDO TB 8.0MM,32FR	10	BX	24.56	8	8	10	20	20	20	20	8	20	20	4	10	12	429	9	11
29772-010	PH SHAVE PREP TRAY W/SPONGES	8	CS	35.68	16	8	8	8	16	16	16	96	48	96	16	48	60	427	30	8
47095-025	3M TIE-ON SURGICAL MASK	48	BX	6.87	48	95	48	48	95	96	1	24	16	48	48	48	13	422	30	27
4121	SOFNET CLEANERS MED DISPENSIN	10	CS	37.27	20	20	10	10	12	24	24	12	12	12	24	0	16	413	8	9
30174-060	3M STERI-DRAPES 17-5/8X35-3/8	1	BX	25.86	12	24	12	16	16	24	24	24	12	24	16	0	16	409	6	10
41-130	ALUM CRUTCH W/STAN SAFE-T-SET	36	PR	11.37	36	35	36	36	36	60	36	36	36	24	26	0	36	405	18	18
5144	DERMICEL HYPO-ALLERGENIC CLOT	36	BX	6.23	36	108	36	72	72	96	48	96	48	96	96	96	63	392	32	28
7747	SAFE-T-WALKER, ADULT	10	EA	33.08	10	10	20	10	10	10	12	12	10	10	8	12	12	380	6	8
30020-040	S/O/P CYSTO PACK 380 STERILE	3	CS	51.59	6	6	9	9	9	6	6	6	6	6	6	6	7	348	3	5
5145	DERMICEL HYPO-ALLERGENIC CLOT	36	BX	6.23	36	72	36	72	72	36	72	108	72	36	43	24	54	336	29	25
13554-010	AMER URI-TOTE URINAL,SHRNK WR	6	CS	33.80	12	12	6	6	13	12	6	12	6	12	12	6	11	323	6	8
30015-020	S/O/P PERI PACK 175 STERILE	2	CS	53.83	8	8	8	8	4	4	4	6	6	6	6	4	6	322	3	5
17060-363	PRESSURE/MONITRNG TUBING 36"TUB	36	BX	6.23	10	5	10	10	10	6	12	10	12	10	16	6	6	316	5	5
11202-020	AMER DUO-THERM DISP PAD,14X20	5	BX	49.20	5	5	8	8	8	6	9	12	9	6	0	6	19	303	5	7
10113-050	TMC SPEEDI BAND ID-URA-8BX/CS	8	BX	34.20	8	8	8	12	14	10	10	10	10	6	6	6	9	296	5	5
11428	TOMAC PERSONAL ICE PACK,28X/C	12	CS	65.50	3	0	3	8	3	0	4	3	3	3	3	4	5	294	3	5
564533542	EPIDURAL TRAY	12	CS	96.70	5	12	10	4	4	0	0	2	12	2	4	4	3	290	2	3
71228-010	GENT-L-KARE SITZ BATH,WHITE	4	CS	35.40	8	8	8	4	4	8	8	4	8	8	4	4	7	283	5	5
29842-010	PH SKIN SCRUB TRAY W/SPNGBGLV	4	CS	38.52	8	2	8	2	4	4	8	5	12	4	5	5	8	269	4	6
47315-130	SHLD BOUF NURSES CAP -REG FLO	2	CS	100.68	2	4	8	2	2	4	5	5	5	5	5	0	18	251	6	6
25996-014	SELF SEALING PCH,7-1/2X14-1/2	4	BX	28.50	2	2	2	2	2	4	8	8	6	8	8	8	19	228	5	3
40-130	ALUM CRUTCH W/STD SAFE-T-SETS	3	PR	11.37	0	12	8	8	12	4	4	8	8	4	0	4	5	204	6	6
30430-060	TYCO VEL CU,PRECAL-ADULT	15	EA	10.39	0	30	10	36	24	24	0	24	36	0	0	0	18	203	13	11
8513	STERI-PAD GAUZE 2" X 2" 100'S	2	DZ	43.23	30	32	4	10	4	0	4	4	28	0	6	6	19	194	11	11
10356-010	PATIENTS BELONGING BAG 5BX/CS	5	BX	37.82	6	4	4	4	4	5	5	2	4	6	6	0	6	184	3	5
22816-130	PH EXAM GLOVES-IND PACK - MED	10	BX	10.52	20	10	10	30	10	10	10	30	20	5	5	0	18	184	13	11
1529-010	PHARM-AIDE FLUID DISPEN SYSTE	3	CS	61.60	3	3	3	3	3	4	4	2	1	2	0	0	3	169	2	3

LAST MONTH	2 MONTHS AGO	3 MONTHS AGO	4 MONTHS AGO	5 MONTHS AGO	6 MONTHS AGO	7 MONTHS AGO	8 MONTHS AGO	9 MONTHS AGO	10 MONTHS AGO	11 MONTHS AGO	12 MONTHS AGO

SEE LAST PAGE FOR TOTAL PURCHASES

Capital equipment acquisition

Charles C. Crider
Director
Materials Management Department
Jess Parrish Memorial Hospital
Titusville, Florida

HOSPITALS ARE spending more on capital equipment purchases today than ever before. The CIT Corporation, a market research firm, surveyed 313 hospitals and found that U.S. hospitals, on an average, spent $536,483 on capital equipment in 1981 as compared with $467,899 in 1980, or 15 percent more in 1981 than in 1980. Nongovernment hospitals participating in the survey purchased an average of $600,296 in capital equipment in 1981, up from $493,226 in 1980—an increase of 22 percent. Governmental and other hospitals paid out $460,195 in 1981, up from $436,903 in 1980—an increase of 5 percent.

KEEPING IN STEP

Speakers at a recent meeting of the Health Lawyers Association in Washington estimated that hospitals will have to come up with $130 billion in the 1980s to finance capital requirements. The author's research suggests that approximately 28 percent of these funds will go for hospital expansion, approximately 67 percent will go for renovation and approximately 5 percent will go for modernization.

According to Valiante, there is a demand among hospitals for renovation. New construction has been postponed in the past several years because of cost containment pressures, high interest rates and unfavorable reimbursement changes. Valiante cited the aging of the population, population migration and the need to upgrade equipment made obsolete by improved technology.

Because of this rapid change in technology, hospitals are having to spend more and more each year to maintain a state-of-the-art status. They are adding new services in an effort to attract new physicians to their community or to entice existing physicians to use their facility. More attention is being placed on new technology as it becomes available, and hospitals will make a concentrated effort to purchase it. By purchasing such technology, each hospital hopes to become unique in the marketplace. Some hospitals have begun to look for, and are considering, ways to expand sophisticated services and projects at off-site locations.

GETTING INVOLVED

The need to purchase capital equipment is likely to continue to increase, and materiel managers must prepare to accept the responsibilities for those purchases. The materiel manager can help ensure that the purchase of capital equipment is cost effective and that the best choice is made to meet the needs of the hospital.

The materiel manager's role in the acquisition of capital equipment varies from hospital to hospital. In some smaller hospitals, the materiel manager's only involvement may be to place the order. Processing is done by the requesting department and the administrative staff. The request filters to the materiel manager, and it is assumed that all information on the request is accurate. This method is not advantageous to the hospital. For the materiel manager to assist in saving money in the purchase of capital equipment, he or she must be involved in the decision-making process as early as possible.

Choosing the best capital equipment also requires time for research that would enable the materiel manager to make a sound recommendation to the administrative staff. To make this recommendation, the materiel manager should investigate several companies that manufacture similar equipment.

Frequently, the equipment requested may not be the best acquisition for the hospital. It is the author's experience that personnel tend to request equipment that is familiar to them or that they have used previously. The materiel manager who has been involved from the beginning knows how the equipment is to be used and can save the hospital valuable dollars.

Most capital equipment comes in a variety of models, and each model will vary according to its functions. Most sales representatives like to promote their top-of-the-line equipment even though such equipment may not be needed. Unless it is known that the additional functions will be utilized in the future, the equipment that is purchased should cover the needs of the department and have the flexibility for future growth, but no more. The dollars saved could be used toward the purchase of other equipment. Materiel managers can facilitate the purchase of capital equipment if they will communicate and plan, implement an equipment review committee and use a team concept.

COMMUNICATING AND PLANNING

The purchase of capital equipment requires communication with the requesting department and time to plan for the acquisition. Good, positive communication can save the materiel manager valuable time. It is not enough to say what is wanted; the materiel manager must follow through on the request to get the desired results. Communication is never simple. Communicating through written policies and procedures is not enough to stop errors. When the purchase of capital equipment is requested in writing, it is very easy to omit information.

Over the years, an unwritten law has maintained that if errors are made, the materiel management department will find them and make the necessary corrections. If the materiel manager has not been involved and knows very little about the equipment, those errors may not be caught. The end result might be receiving equipment that cannot be used.

Errors are costly to the requesting department and to the hospital. To the user, it means a loss of time before the equipment can be put into service and a loss of productivity. To the hospital, it could mean a loss of a cash discount if a delay in payment to the supplier occurs, additional costs in shipping fees if the equipment has to be returned and the possibility of a restocking fee. Through

good communication, such errors can be reduced.

IMPLEMENTING EQUIPMENT REVIEW

To assist the materiel manager in planning for capital equipment acquisitions, an equipment review committee may be established. At Jess Parrish Memorial Hospital, it consists of members of the medical staff, administration, nursing administration, plant operations and clinical equipment and is chaired by the materiel manager. Other hospital personnel may be invited to the meeting, depending on the equipment to be purchased. For example, if laboratory equipment is being purchased, the chief laboratory medical technologist is invited to the meeting.

An equipment review committee can discuss the equipment in detail, thus enabling the materiel manager to know exactly what is needed. Through this committee, a checklist can be made that will assure the materiel manager that all questions are covered before the equipment is purchased. It also will ensure that equipment purchased can be used throughout the hospital. The checklist should include the following:

1. Service: Who will do the service, and how long will it take to receive it? Is there an emergency number for service after normal working hours and on holidays, and is there an additional cost for such service?
2. Maintenance: Is a preventive maintenance agreement offered?
3. Warranty: What is the length of the warranty, and what is covered (parts, labor and travel time)?

4. Delivery time: How long will it take to receive the equipment, and who pays the freight?
5. Special requirements
   - physical dimensions and the location of utility connections;
   - utility connections required (electrical, gas, water, steam, air, oxygen or drain);
   - connected ventilations or exhaust;
   - environmental operating requirements, operating temperature range, required humidity range or special lighting;
   - heat generated by the equipment; and
   - special electrical characteristics such as dedicated circuits.

USING A TEAM CONCEPT

Once the equipment needs of the requesting department have been determined, negotiations for the equipment should follow. A negotiations team is not always easy to create. Frequently, personal-

---

Frequently, personalities and titles stand in the way of successful negotiations.

---

ities and titles stand in the way of successful negotiations. Some materiel managers expect other department directors to approach them. In the best interests of the hospital, the materiel manager may have to take the first step. Once that first step has been initiated, the rest will fall into place. The old saying that "two heads are better than one" applies in hospitals. Materiel

managers need the technical expertise of the using department, and users need materiel managers' expertise in purchasing practices.

For years, manufacturers have successfully used the team concept to their advantage. Often, when it is time to purchase a costly piece of equipment and a meeting is called with the manufacturer, the salesperson, his or her manager and a "specialist" attend the negotiations. Materiel managers have been no match for such well-planned sales teams. But if they create their own team, they will be in a position to negotiate a better price for the hospital. Good communication and the creation of a team are musts if materiel managers are to stand their ground.

Selecting a leader

To assist in effective negotiations with the manufacturer, the team must first meet to plan a strategy. A leader must be selected to direct the discussion. This may or may not be the materiel manager. If someone else can do it better, then that person should be selected. Dual leadership is another possibility, depending on the areas of discussion. For example, if the discussion evolves around technical aspects, a team member who uses the equipment should assume the leader's role. If the discussion evolves around service, delivery or warranty, the materiel manager should assume the leader's role. The main objective is getting the best price for the equipment.

Once a leader has been selected, it is that person's responsibility to ensure that the team's plan is kept in order and that the team does not get sidetracked. The team should be prepared to really listen to what the manufacturer is saying. Care should be taken that, with an organized plan, the team does not get so involved that it does not hear the other side. It is important to be prepared to make some concessions, but to also know in advance what those concessions are and not deviate. This may call for another meeting, so that other concessions, not previously agreed to, can be discussed and accepted or rejected.

Keeping calm

Team members must be careful in not only what they say but how they say it. If tempers are allowed to go unchecked and a heated discussion is allowed, no one benefits. If comments or threats that the manufacturer cannot accept are made, the end result could be having to purchase a piece of equipment that was the second choice. No one wins in that type of situation. There is no place for hot tempers on a negotiation team.

Members should always strive to maintain a professional attitude. They have the right to tell a supplier how they feel or if they have had problems with his or her company in the past, but care should be taken in how those views are expressed. Alienation is not the objective. Attitude and tone of voice will set the stage for later discussions. Equipment negotiations cannot always be in the hospital's favor. Manufacturers do not stay in business by giving away equipment. A final price should be acceptable and fair to all parties concerned.

MEETING THE CHALLENGES

If the prediction that $130 billion will be needed to finance capital equipment in the 1980s is correct, then materiel managers have busy years ahead. They should continue to accept the challenges that these acquisitions will bring. With good communication and planning, through the implementation of an equipment review committee, and the use of a team concept, capital equipment can be acquired more easily.

Procurement of major equipment

Steven R. Campbell
Director of Materiel
Coronado Hospital
Coronado, California

DEVELOPMENTS in medical technology are creating a new series of demands in the area of the procurement of capital equipment for health care institutions. The acquisition of this equipment requires that substantial amounts of money be expended for a single purchase, and the final cost of the equipment (including actual cost, freight, service contracts, installation, disposition of used equipment, special insurance costs, and special training costs) is more difficult to evaluate and negotiate than, say, the final cost of medical supplies. These difficulties are, however, providing an excellent opportunity for demonstrating to administration that the procurement of capital equipment requires the kind of expertise that only a person in a materiel function can provide.

WHAT IS CAPITAL EQUIPMENT?

Capital equipment may be regarded as the fixed assets of a hospital, the cost of which is more properly charged to a capital account than to expense. Such assets are essential "durable" or "capital" goods that are purchased for either direct use by the hospital (fixtures, desks, computer systems, etc.) or direct patient care (ranging from a scale to a computerized axial tomography [CAT] scanner). This leads to a useful classification in the two divisions of multipurpose and single-purpose equipment.[1]

Multipurpose equipment may have a variety of uses, may be used in several hospitals, tends to have a longer life, and may have considerable salvage value. Shelving, certain classes of computers, and standard typewriters are typical examples. Single-purpose equipment, ranging from operating tables to intensive care unit (ICU) beds to arthroscopy equipment, is designed for a limited number of purposes. Because of this the purchaser's specifications usually require extensive consultation between the purchasing staff and the technical staff, which might include administration, the medical and nursing staff, and engineering. It is single-purpose rather than multipurpose equipment that should receive higher priority in terms of the purchasing agent's time and expertise.

FROM CHALLENGES TO OPPORTUNITIES

The procurement of capital equipment offers special challenges to the materiel manager. These, in turn, offer valuable opportunities to demonstrate skill in an area where cost savings can be monumental.

Financial planning

First, the acquisition of equipment usually requires that substantial amounts of money be expended for a single purpose. This may require a special form of financing, such as an installment plan or a lease plan. Sound knowledge of alternatives in the area of financing gives the materiel manager an edge in negotiation. Special methods of financing might include the following:

1. By the vendor under an established short- or long-range installment plan;
2. By outside sources, such as loans from financial institutions; and
3. By a rental agreement with a financial institution, which may provide for the application of rental payments to the price.[2] This may actually prove to be a leasing agreement (to be discussed later).

Obviously the financial officer of the hospital is responsible for reaching decisions in the area of purchasing capital equipment. However various possibilities known to the materiel manager should be called to the officer's attention.

Long-term savings

Second, the final cost of equipment is more difficult to determine with exactness than is the final cost of medical supplies. The initial cost of equipment is only a part of the total cost, which at best can only be estimated. This may include, but is not limited to, the effects of idle time, obsolescence, maintenance and repair, and direct operating cost. More important, the cost of supplies to be used with the equipment should always be considered. The materiel management department at Coronado

Hospital was asked to evaluate two infusion pumps. Although the cost of one unit was significantly less, the cassettes cost almost twice as much, and it was decided that the more expensive model would be purchased because of long-range savings.

The income to be derived should also be taken into account. A factor in determining whether to buy a piece of equipment can be the length of time that it will take for the equipment to "pay for itself."[3]

As a general rule an investment in equipment made to improve efficiency or to increase the patient census should pay for itself in four to five years. This criterion is roughly comparable to that used by profit-making organizations. The "payback" range depends on the financial condition of the hospital. A hospital in good financial condition might allow for the equipment to take a longer time to pay for itself. A hospital in a less stable financial condition might require a period of less than four years. This needs to be discussed with the financial officer.

The savings that may be considered in making this kind of evaluation can be, but certainly is not limited to, the areas of human resources, increased patient census, and better working conditions.

Will a new piece of equipment require fewer employees? This is where most savings occur because a large investment is more easily justified if even one employee can be taken off the payroll or transferred to another department. It is important to make sure, however, that this savings does not simply mean longer coffee breaks for the existing staff.

When a capital acquisition, such as an ophthalmic microscope for a hospital that has never specialized in ophthalmology

means that more patients will be admitted to the institution, purchasing the equipment should be seriously considered. It should first be determined, however, that the physician intends to bring more patients to the institution as a result of the availability of the equipment.

Although better working conditions are a difficult parameter to measure in terms of actual savings, many studies have shown that a comfortable working environment (relative to equipment, such as room dividers, upgraded typewriters, etc.) increases the efficiency of the employees and ultimately saves money.

Broadened scope

There is a third challenge that offers the materiel manager an opportunity to demonstrate the importance and value of the relatively new field of materiel management in health care. Because of the comparatively long life and the investment involved, equipment items, particularly major ones, are likely to be bought less frequently than other types of purchases, and as a result the stakes are higher. This is because the purchase of major equipment often commits the hospital to a series of other comparatively permanent decisions, such as instituting a new medical procedure.

The materiel manager, with administrative support, is in a key position to influence the selection of this equipment. This is because the position's sphere of influence can and should affect every department in the hospital, not just the department requesting the equipment. The materiel management function, which is in the process of development, no longer focuses on purchasing alone, but is also evolving into a liaison between the administration and financial departments, and the rest of the hospital in equipment acquisition.

HOSPITAL POLICY

Because of the unique nature and expense of capital acquisition, a policy is necessary for all departments of the hospital. The following discussion outlines a policy that has proven helpful and efficient.

Approximately three months before the beginning of the next fiscal year, all departments, while making budgets for that year, need to specify the capital equipment needed, and divide it into two groups: medical and nonmedical. These are submitted to administration and ultimately the board of directors for review and approval.

After this approval, administration and materiel management will discuss the nonmedical equipment with the respective department heads and compile a prioritized list, setting a projected date of purchase for each item. The medical equipment is discussed by a technical services committee composed of three or more representatives from the medical staff and administration, and the materiel manager. This committee discusses the capital requirements (as listed on the budgets) with each department head in a series of meetings. A priority list of equipment results from these meetings, and a projected date of purchase for each item is scheduled. The committee continues to meet once a month to reset priorities as it deems necessary. It also discusses medical

equipment that has not been budgeted but has been requested by a physician.

The materiel manager then compiles a list of all proposed capital expenditures for the fiscal year and meets monthly with the financial officer to review the cash flow of the hospital. As monies become available, the department head requesting the equipment is asked to review again that department's need for the equipment. If it is decided that the equipment is still a necessity, an equipment requisition is submitted to the department of materiel management for negotiation of price, terms of service, warranties, etc.

If the equipment coming up for purchase according to the aforementioned list is over a certain amount (from $5,000 to $20,000 according to the policy of the hospital), the administrator refers the documentation and recommendations to the executive finance committee. Then upon approval it is presented to the board of directors. If approved by the board the actual purchasing process begins. If not the administrator seeks another resolution to the matter.

INVOLVEMENT OF OTHER DEPARTMENTS

Because of the nature of capital equipment, procurement usually involves more departments than the one requesting its purchase; administration, finance, and engineering are also directly involved.

A form such as that shown in Figure 1 may be used to request a piece of equipment. It should include the information required for the proper decision to be made and may be used with the procurement procedure.

EQUIPMENT PURCHASE REQUISITION

No. 000855

TABLE A

TO BE COMPLETED BY REQUESTING DEPARTMENT

NAME OF ITEM

DESCRIPTION

QUANTITY WANTED	MODEL/CATALOG NUMBER	WAS THIS ON THIS YEARS BUDGET	EST. LIFE
			YRS
EQUIPMENT BEING REPLACED		CONDITION AND AGE	
ADDITIONAL SUPPLIES NEEDED TO OPERATE THIS ITEM		MONTHLY USAGE	COST/MO. $
JUSTIFICATION FOR REQUEST			

REQUESTING DEPARTMENT	SUPERVISOR	DATE	DEPARTMENT HEAD	DATE

TO BE COMPLETED BY PURCHASING DEPARTMENT

VENDOR   ADDRESS

SPECIFICATIONS

UNIT COST $	TOTAL COST $	DISCOUNT	SALVAGE VALUE REPLACED ITEM $	DELIVERY TIME DAYS	GUARANTEE MOS	EST. LIFE YRS

REMARKS

	PURCHASING AGENT	DATE

TO BE COMPLETED BY ENGINEERING DEPARTMENT

INSTALLATION COST	INSTALLATION AND TESTING TIME	REMOVAL COST OF REPLACED ITEM	REMOVAL TIME

REMARKS

	CHIEF ENGINEER	DATE

ADMINISTRATIVE ACTION

DATE

☐ APPROVED   ☐ NOT APPROVED   ☐ RETURNED MORE INFORMATION NEEDED

REMARKS

GOVERNING BOARD	DATE	ADMINISTRATOR	DATE

PURCHASING DEPARTMENT ACTION

DATE ORDERED	P.O. NO.	ORDER PLACED BY	DELIVERY DATE

#4 PCH

DEPT. ORDERING

Figure 1. Equipment purchase requisition.

Major participants

Because administration is ultimately responsible for achieving improvements in patient care and for realizing cost and profit objectives, it is generally open to better methods or better quality, and for

---

It is important that the materiel manager be thoroughly knowledgeable about developments that will enable the hospital to offer patients the kind of care that the administration strives to provide.

---

replacement of obsolete and unsafe equipment. Because administrators have the final say on whether or not a piece of equipment will be acquired, it is important that the materiel manager be thoroughly knowledgeable about new developments

that will enable the hospital to offer patients the kind of care that the administration strives to provide. (See boxed material.)

The finance department is involved with all capital equipment planning and procurement because it must determine the best way to finance the capital investment, as well as the effect the purchase will have on cash flow. It is important that the materiel manager be kept aware of the hospital's continually changing cash flow, especially in a smaller institution, since cash flow ultimately determines if, when, and how a piece of equipment will be purchased.

The engineering department plays an important part in capital acquisition, so it is essential that materiel management and engineering work together in the evaluation, planning, receipt, warranty, and safety compliance stages of many equipment purchases.

Checklist for Equipment Acquisition

1. Develop a list of equipment (both medical and nonmedical) requested by various departments.
2. Work with administration, a technical services committee, and each department to arrange the list in terms of priorities.
3. When it is time to acquire a piece of equipment, evaluate the following parameters.
   - How is the equipment to be financed? Lease or Buy?
   - What will the "final" cost of the equipment be after a given time (two years, five years, etc.)?
   - What kind of savings (if any) will be enjoyed by the hospital?
   - What kind of increase in patient census will be enjoyed?
   - What effect will the equipment have on personnel requirements?
   - How will the equipment affect working conditions?
   - How involved should the engineering department be in this purchase?
4. Enter into negotiation to determine contractual terms:
   - Pricing;
   - Installation;
   - Specifications regarding codes and standards;
   - Operating manuals;
   - Back orders;
   - Final receipt and examination;
   - Warranties;
   - Recalls;
   - Return of faulty equipment;
   - Inservice training; and
   - Engineering service.

Seethaler recommends that engineering be consulted only before buying equipment designated as "technical."[4] He defines "technical" as requiring a utility hookup (electrical, steam, gas, water, air, or other), and he believes engineering should be consulted when acquiring this type of equipment because it can help write specifications for complex purchases. This consultation and approval may be confirmed on the equipment purchase requisition. (See Figure 1.)

Maintenance questions

The form shown in the Appendix may be used by materiel management and engineering to obtain information regarding market conditions, warranty and service, installation, and inservice programs before the purchase is made. Receipts for technical equipment should be held for maintenance review after the purchase. Operating manuals, schematics, and warranty data should be distributed to the local and master file systems before equipment is installed.

There are additional benefits of open dialogue with maintenance. It can result in service and repair records that assist in cost benefits or a justification analysis of new systems. Technical review of existing equipment maintenance-history and operating characteristics can also preclude unauthorized cannibalization and attendant liabilities.

FINANCING OF THE PURCHASE

Before any commitment to buy a major item is given approval, careful thought should be given not only to the desirability of the purchase but also to the means of payment. Regardless of what else may be said for the equipment, unless it can be paid for, no action can be taken.

Buying

When the budget is initially set up for the coming fiscal year, it is advantageous to provide for two types of capital expenditures. The first type covers probable expenditures that, although properly chargeable to some capital account, are still too small to be brought directly to the technical services committee or administration. These would be mainly replacement items, such as instruments, parts, desks, and standard typewriters. A limit on the cost of each piece of requested equipment should be fixed to include these items, such as $200 to $500.

The second type includes larger expenditures that are also provided for in the budget. At times acquiring enough capital to purchase more costly equipment is a problem, especially in the present market of tight money supply and high interest rates.

Leasing

As a result, there has been significant movement toward leasing, either through the equipment manufacturer, a third party leasing specialist, or a financial house. Leasing is a dynamic and growing enterprise. In the past 20 years it has enjoyed phenomenal growth and is now a multi-billion-dollar business.

What to ask

The scope of this article does not allow a discussion of the two main types of leases (one financial and the other operational) except to say that the materiel manager must exercise utmost care in passing judgment on leasing and the lessor. It should be asked, is the lessor:

- Fair and reasonable in dealings with customers?;
- Financially strong?; and
- If a sole source, prone to be arbitrary in the periodic adjustment of rental and other fees?

Leasing advocates point out that the concept of leasing involves payments for the use of the equipment rather than payment for the privilege of owning the equipment. There are no cut and dried answers as to leasing's advantages and disadvantages. There are, however, fundamental aspects of leasing with which every materiel manager and financial administrator should be familiar.

Pros and cons

The main advantages are:

1. The risk of obsolescence can be minimized or eliminated. Many pieces of medical equipment can be negotiated so that the lessor will provide the latest and most sophisticated models.
2. Maintenance problems can be eliminated or substantially reduced.
3. Because of the availability of monies, leasing provides a wider range of options to the hospital.
4. The burden of investment is shifted from the hospital to the supplier or lessee. This means that the institution's working capital can be used for other needs.
5. Leasing can permit a new procedure to be instituted at the hospital even though the capital funds necessary to purchase the needed equipment are

not available at the time. This is especially helpful when a new specialist joins the staff and a large amount of capital is initially needed to obtain equipment.

The disadvantages of leasing are:

1. It is almost always more expensive than an outright purchase, and will usually be more expensive than other methods of financing.
2. In some types of leases, the hospital may be somewhat restricted in the control and use of the equipment.
3. Other disadvantages can materialize, depending on the actual terms negotiated in the lease contract. The hospital must, therefore, see that the contract does not result in any restrictive or otherwise negative conditions being placed on it.[5]

PROCUREMENT BY NEGOTIATION

Procurement begins after all of the departments have been contacted and the necessary approvals have been given. Housley states that the more specific the written understandings concerning the equipment being procured are, the better the purchase.[6] He recommends that the hospital's regular purchase order procedure be used and that a list of supplemental considerations, preferably signed by the authorized representatives, be made an addendum to the purchase order.

Art and craft

These considerations often are or should be the result of negotiation. Procurement by negotiation is an art. Its goal is to arrive at a common understanding through bargaining on the essentials of a contract, such as delivery, specifications, price, and terms. Artistic skill is required because all of the factors involved are interrelated, and a combination of judgment, tact, and common sense is necessary to negotiate a contract that will benefit the hospital and the vendor. The effective negotiator is always attuned to the possibilities and alternatives in bargaining with the vendor. Only through an acute awareness of relative bargaining strength is a negotiator able to know where to use firmness or where concessions may be made.

Negotiation may be considered the psychology of persuasion, and nothing contributes more toward successful negotiations than advance planning of objectives and strategy. The materiel manager should enter the session with a positive attitude toward achieving planned objectives, as well as having decided on the maximum extent of potential concessions. All pertinent facts should be collected and studied before the meeting so that the buyer will be ready to answer promptly and speak with determination on any counterpoints the vendor may present.

Rules of the game

Aljian[7] recommends that the following tactics be avoided:
1. Trying to prove the vendor is wrong (while the materiel manager may win the point, in most cases the vendor will not reduce the price);
2. Getting so buried in details that the objectives are lost; and
3. Conceding any point early in the negotiations.

Often a vendor's fear of losing a hospital's business, especially if the hospital has done business with that vendor for a relatively long time, will bring greater concessions.

According to Aljian, the materiel manager should practice the following tactics:
1. Negotiate at the hospital and not on the vendor's territory.
2. Negotiate with those representatives who have the authority to make concessions, the kind of concessions that can only be obtained from higher levels of management.
3. Remain silent at times. Often a vendor's fear of losing a hospital's business, especially if the hospital has done business with that vendor for a relatively long time, will bring greater concessions.
4. Keep the target in mind and know beforehand what gains can be expected through negotiation.
5. Plan ahead with the hospital's negotiating team.
6. Negotiate for long-term concessions. A piece of equipment costing $10,000 but with a service contract of $3,000 a year is a lot more expensive over the long run than a piece of equipment costing $13,000 with a service contract of $5,000 a year.
7. Be careful regarding the facts. It can be disconcerting for materiel managers to have the wrong information.
8. If the talks hit a snag, call for a break.

9. Enlist the aid of specialists from engineering, finance, the requesting department, and any other department involved to help evaluate the benefits of the equipment and contract.
10. Always be fair.

WHAT IS NEGOTIABLE?

It is common knowledge that the actual cost of a piece of medical equipment (excluding transportation, service contracts, and installation) is fixed in many cases. This is especially true when dealing with a piece of equipment that is manufactured by only one company. What then should be considered in the negotiating process? The following discussion presents the particulars offered by Housley.[8]

It should be made clear that the price indicated on the purchase order will be the hospital's total financial commitment for a purchase. Any additional parts or accessories that may be needed to install the equipment and make it operative will be at the expense of the supplying company unless otherwise stated in writing.

Many companies will request a partial payment arrangement, but the materiel manager should make it clear that it is hospital policy to pay total invoice price only upon installation and acceptance of the equipment, and that no other payment schedule is acceptable. This policy not only speeds up the delivery, but also gives the hospital interest on the money for a longer time.

All equipment specified and quoted should meet or exceed all of the necessary city, state, and federal standards, and have Underwriters' Laboratories (UL) approval where applicable. All equipment will be inspected upon receipt by a biomedical engineer or other responsible party and, if found in violation of the delineated specifications, will be returned freight collect.

Operating manuals, pertinent electrical and mechanical schematics, and current parts list must be received before payment of the invoice. All equipment must be shipped at the same time. This negates the possibility of partial shipments and the likelihood of storage loss. If there is a back order of a part or accessory, it is better that the company and not the hospital receive and be responsible for it.

A company representative should be responsible for the final equipment receipt checklist before installation and should determine from quality and quantity standpoints that the specified equipment has arrived and is ready for installation. The company selected should be responsible for detailing instructions for equipment layout and installation. This includes specifications for equipment arrangement and the necessary completion details for meeting such requirements as electrical needs.

All equipment or parts thereof must carry at least a one-year full warranty on parts and labor, endorsed and supported in writing by the manufacturer or distributor. Many companies adhere to a list price but are open to negotiating the length of the warranty. Materiel management should aim for a two-year warranty, and if this cannot be accomplished should settle for a cost-reduced maintenance contract. In addition there is much to be accomplished in the negotiation of a five- or six-year price-protected maintenance contract at the time of the purchase. (It should be kept in mind that the hospital's clout exists *before* the purchase is made.)

The hospital purchase order number

must appear on all pertinent cartons, packages, packing lists, and invoices. There must also be clarification as to the responsibility of the vendor in cases of equipment or attachment recall. The total cost of the recall should be borne by the manufacturer. If the equipment or part thereof must be returned to the manufacturer because of a fault of the company, it should be at the company's expense. A qualified representative of the company should provide the necessary inservice education to all appropriate hospital personnel.

ENGINEERING SERVICE

Most sellers of major medical equipment maintain a continuing interest in their equipment after it is sold and installed. Technical sales service, especially in the electromedical field, is provided by a vendor to a potential hospital to determine the designs and specifications of the equipment believed best-suited to the particular requirements of the hospital, and also to ensure that once bought, the equipment functions properly. Most vendors of electromedical equipment believe that their equipment is so technologically advanced that none but their own biomedical engineers can either install the equipment or service it. Service of this type is

often highly recommended, especially in a smaller hospital, which, in the probable absence of a fulltime biomedical engineer or an external certified biomedical repair facility, may need such assistance.

In larger hospitals, however, it is quite profitable for the materiel manager to work closely with the maintenance department in evaluating available service arrangements. Seethaler reduced service contract requirements in frequency and contingency by having his department work with the bioengineering department and maintenance department.[9]

Seethaler states that the majority of calls for service are now channeled through purchasing, biomedical, or maintenance personnel. Readily identifiable problems are corrected and the equipment is checked out by biomedical personnel and placed back in service. More complicated problems are identified, if possible, and the service agent is notified of a needed repair.

The procurement of capital equipment requires that materiel managers "do their homework" by studying all of the parameters involved. Although a great deal of study and evaluation are sometimes necessary when making a capital purchase, the payoff in terms of monies saved and other benefits to the hospital can be tremendous.

REFERENCES

1. England, W. and Leenders, M. *Purchasing and Materials Management* (Homewood, Ill.: Richard D. Irwin, Inc. 1975) p. 713.

2. Aljian, G. *Purchasing Handbook* (McGraw-Hill 1973) p. 17-26.

3. Ammer, D. "Purchasing Pointers." *Hospital Purchasing Management* 4:3 (March 1979) p. 9-10.

4. Seethaler, M. "Materials Management and Mainte-

nance: Partners in Cost Containment." *Hospital Purchasing Management* 4:6 (June 1979) p. 11-14.

5. Aljian, G. *Purchasing Handbook* p. 15-17.

6. Housley, C. *Hospital Materiel Management* (Germantown, Md.: Aspen Systems Corp. 1978) p. 219-220.

7. Aljian, G. *Purchasing Handbook* p. 9-11.

8. Housley, C. *Hospital Materiel Management* p. 219-220.

9. Seethaler, M. "Materials Management and Maintenance." p. 11-14.

Appendix
Vendor's checklist— capital equipment

Note: This form will be referenced in any purchase order issued under this request for proposal. Answer all applicable questions to the best of your ability.

I. *PRICE: MARKET CONDITIONS*

    A. Your price will remain firm for: _____ days.

    B. What is List Price? _____

    C. When do you expect your next price increase to occur? _____.

    D. What do you expect the increase to be? _____ (Amount or Percent)

II. *WARRANTY-SERVICE*

    A. What is the warranty period on this equipment? _____ months

    B. When does warranty period begin? _____

    C. Who will service this equipment during the warranty period? _____

    D. Do you have service contracts on this equipment? ( ) Yes   ( ) No
        1. Current annual cost? _____
        2. What is the point of origin of service? _____
        3. What is the anticipated response time to our facility? _____

    E. Do you offer a training program for our repair technicians? ( ) Yes   ( ) No

    F. Does this equipment meet the current and applicable requirement or codes of the following:
        1. Occupational Safety & Health Act   ( ) Yes   ( ) No
        2. Underwriters' Laboratory   ( ) Yes   ( ) No
        3. National Fire Protection Association   ( ) Yes   ( ) No

    G. List special tool or equipment requirement to perform preventive and/or repair maintenance to this equipment: _____.

III. *INSTALLATION*

    A. Will installation be the responsibility of: ( ) Vendor   ( ) Medical Center? Is there an additional cost involved? ( ) Yes   ( ) No
If yes, state cost $_____.

    B. Upon receipt of equipment, will your personnel set up the equipment according to the manufacturer's specifications? ( ) Yes   ( ) No
If No, Explain: _____ .

    C. Are there utility requirements?
        1. Electrical Voltage: _____ Amperage: _____
        2. Drains: ( ) Yes _____
           Water: ( ) Yes _____
           Other: ( ) Yes _____
           Specifics: _____ .

    D. Will this equipment have all necessary mechanical, electrical trim or other appurtenances for use upon its arrival? ( ) Yes   ( ) No
If No, what needs to be done? _____

    E. Will any site preparation be necessary? ( ) Yes   ( ) No
If Yes, explain: _____ .

    F. Are there supplies necessary for utilization of this equipment?
( ) Yes   ( ) No
If Yes, explain what, from whom, and suggest start-up supply.

        _____
        _____

    G. Is a start-up supply included in the price of the equipment? ( ) Yes   ( ) No
If so, what: _____ .

    H. Who uncrates the equipment and what must occur upon delivery? _____
        _____ .

    I. Will this equipment require any unloading equipment to make safe receipt at time of delivery? ( ) Yes   ( ) No
If Yes, specify: _____ .

    J. If installation is involved, will you coordinate delivery and installation to take place on the same date as a term of the Purchase Order? ( ) Yes   ( ) No
Explain: _____ .

IV. *INSERVICE AND USE*

    A. Do you provide a unit for in-house demonstration or Trial and Evaluation?
( ) Yes   ( ) No
If Yes, specify and state any terms: _____ .

    B. If this equipment is used to perform a patient chargeable service, what is the average charge for this service by other Hospitals? $_____ /treatment.

C. Will an upgrade be required/available in the forseeable future? ( ) Yes
( ) No
If Yes, explain: _____ .

D. Will an Inservice on the use of this equipment be required? ( ) Yes ( ) No
If Yes, state full specifics: _____
_____ .

E. How long has this equipment been on the market? _____ Months _____
Years.
List three (3) institutions, preferably in this area, who use this equipment:

INSTITUTION	NAME & TITLE OF USER
1.	
2.	
3.	

V. *VENDOR*

Use this section below to list any additional information which you feel would be of interest to us in making an award decision.

_____
_____
_____
_____
_____

Completed By: _____   Date: _____
Name & Title

A comparative analysis of a cost-plus purchasing system and a pricing service program

George P. Page, R.D.
Director of Food Service
Kenmore Mercy Hospital and Skilled
*   Nursing Facility*
Buffalo, New York

RECOGNIZING the need for prudent buying, area dietary directors under the sponsorship of the Western New York Hospital Association (WNYHA) and Blue Cross of Western New York assembled a committee to explore methods of containing costs without compromising quality or service. The initial meetings in the summer of 1974 were concerned with exploring methods used to procure food.

A cost-plus program was selected for purchasing groceries. The new group purchasing unit determined that this was the most expeditious way to launch a group purchasing venture covering approximately 1,200 grocery items. Prospective grocery vendors were asked to submit bids on a yearly basis, based on a percentage markup over their costs. For instance, the winning bid one year was as follows: canned items and frozen items, 10 percent over cost; fresh meat and dairy products, 8 percent over cost. Cost was defined as the price on the invoice to the vendor plus the freight in.

After three years with the cost-plus program, the committee tried to evaluate the program's effectiveness. It became apparent that there was no feasible way to do this objectively, since there was no basis for comparison with other vendors. In 1978 the WNYHA dropped the cost-plus program and adopted the grocery pricing service which was being used by the Ontario Hospital Association (OHA).

The OHA's group purchasing committee was using a pricing service for purchasing groceries. This system allowed all vendors to submit prices on a monthly basis for all 1,200 grocery items. The items and corresponding prices were sent to each dietary director. This allowed each director to compare prices and select the desired brand. The vendors all received copies of the monthly pricing book, and were able to evaluate their respective positions in the market.

In 1980 a study was made of the effectiveness of the pricing service versus the cost-plus program. A random sample of 50 items was selected and the prices paid in December of each year from 1974 to 1979 were collected from past invoices. The May 1978 prices were also included because that was the last month of the cost-plus program. The Kenmore Mercy Hospital (KMH) prices were indexed using 1974 as the base year, since this was the last year that groceries were purchased without the benefit of a group program. The weights used in the formula were obtained from the WNYHA's data on usage figures submitted by the dietary directors.

The yearly prices with their corresponding weights were fed into the following formula:

$$P = \text{antilog} \frac{\Sigma P_o q_o P_1 / P_o \ 100}{\Sigma P_o q_o}$$

This formula is a weighted geometric mean of price relatives, with P_o equal to the price of product in the base year, q_o equal to the quantity of product used in the base year and P_1 equal to the price of product for the current year being measured. It is more conservative than the arithmetic mean and uses weights from the base period only. It is free of upward or downward bias.

The results were then compared with the corresponding Consumer Price Index (CPI) for each year. (See Table 1.) The results are graphed in Figure 1.

The initial impact of group purchasing

Table 1. Yearly comparison of the two programs to the CPI

Month/year	CPI (food)	CPI % change	KMHI	KMHI % change	Variance %
December 1974	170.0	+12.2	100.0	N/A	N/A
December 1975	181.0	+ 6.5	89.1	− 10.9	+17.4
December 1976	181.9	+ .6	87.6	− 1.7	+ 2.3
December 1977	192.2	+ 8.1	97.8	+11.6	− 3.5
May 1978	204.3	+ 6.3	102.0	+ 4.3	+ 2.0
December 1978	214.2	+ 5.2	100.0	− 2.0	+ 7.2
December 1979	237.1	+10.1	106.8	+ 6.8	+ 3.3

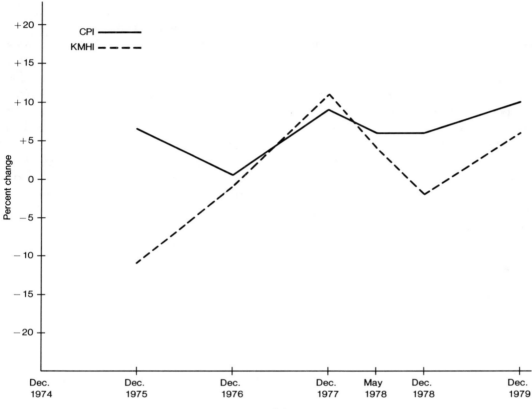

Figure 1. Comparison of the KMHI to the CPI.

is clearly evident in the +17.4 percent net variance at the end of 1975. This emphasized the advantage of group purchasing as a means of effecting cost containment. As one analyzes the figures after 1975, it becomes apparent that the Kenmore Mercy Hospital Index (KMHI) has beaten the CPI in every year except 1977. In the aggregate, however, the KMHI is favorable.

Table 2. Trend analysis results showing KMHI for 1978 and 1979 with the cost-plus program

Year	CPI	CPI % change	KMHI	KMHI % change	Variance %
1978	214.1	+ 5.2	109.1	+ 6.5	1.3
1979	237.1	+10.1	123.2	+11.4	1.3

However, this analysis did not show which program was better in terms of cost containment. Therefore a trend analysis was performed. A linear regression and correlation was performed. The KMHI was regressed on the CPI. The regression was performed on the indices during the cost-plus years. The factor or correlation coefficient proved to be .969. The predictability of the regression analysis is 96.9 percent accurate. The December 1978 and December 1979 CPIs were then regressed on the cost-plus program. A t test was performed on this regression and proved to be within the .05 confidence limit. The results are shown in Table 2.

The result of this trend analysis shows a KMHI of 109.1 for 1980 and 123.2 for 1979. When this is compared with the actual KMHI of 100.0 for 1978 and 106.8 for 1979, one sees a significantly slower rise with the pricing service method than with the cost-plus program.

Therefore it can be concluded that under the cost-plus program, the food would have cost approximately 8.5 percent more in 1978 and 4.6 percent more in 1979.

Hospital capital equipment purchasing in an investor-owned environment

Elbert O. Garner
Assistant Vice President
Materiel Management
Hospital Corporation of America
Nashville, Tennessee

FROM THE VIEWPOINT of the hospital materiel manager, capital equipment purchasing has always been a problem. Who makes the selection as to model and manufacturer? Who negotiates the price and terms? What or who determines the equipment finally selected—price or manufacturer? These and other questions plague the hospital materiel manager, regardless of hospital ownership.

In some investor-owned hospitals, many of these decisions are made at the corporate level. The manufacturer, model and price are finalized at the corporate level. The only thing the hospital materiel manager does is receive the equipment.

Hospital Corporation of America (HCA) has a philosophy of decentralization and strong local autonomy. As a result, capital equipment purchasing in the owned hospitals is divided into two functions: (1) capital equipment purchasing for new construction projects—whether for a completely new hospital or an addition to an existing facility; and (2) capital equipment purchasing for new or additional equipment for an operating hospital.

ACQUISITIONS FOR CONSTRUCTION PROJECTS

For the past 14 years the Materiel Management Department of HCA has experimented with methods of establishing standard equipment lists for construction and renovation of facilities. Among these methods was the prototype list based on bed size, which meant that every 50-bed hospital received the same list of equipment. This method proved inadequate because it failed to take into consideration the various and unique medical practices that exist in different parts of the country.

In 1977 HCA established the position of project equipment manager, which enabled it to have one individual in charge of each project from inception to completion. This allowed the Materiel Management Department to make one-point contact with all individuals at the hospital and solved many of the problems that had existed with previous methods.

Computerized tracking

At the same time, a minicomputer was brought into the department, and a new program was established that is unique in its versatility. Some of the reasons for establishing the computerized system were to allow rapid response to requests from hospitals and to document, in detail, every item that would go into a project, regardless of size.

Within the computer are two basic lists: (1) the space master, which lists every department, every space and every item within that space that the department recommends for the hospital's use in the project; and (2) the item master, which the project equipment manager can use to replace items in the space master that hospital personnel feel are not appropriate for their needs for a particular project. For example, for radiology, the department has three contractual arrangements that can be used, depending on the preference of the radiologist and the service offered in the hospital's geographic area. The flexibility of the system makes the list usable regardless of where the project is located. Because HCA is a decentralized operation, the Materiel Management Department can allow each hospital direct input into its individual project.

The space master list allows the project equipment manager to meet the demands of any size project, from a one-room addition to a 2,000-bed hospital. The system is based on a simple fact—any project can be equipped according to the spaces that will exist in the facility. When the project is broken down into individual spaces, it can be addressed in a simple, yet detailed, fashion. The item master list allows the flexibility to tailor the facility to the needs of the local community. This list is constantly updated and is never permitted to become static.

Diverse talents

The individuals who were brought into the department as project equipment managers have hospital backgrounds that include nursing service, materiel management, respiratory therapy, pharmacy, laboratory and radiology. These individuals not only bring to the department a great degree of expertise within individual areas, but, by working closely together, they can provide constant and valuable support for each project. The HCA believes that the degree of teamwork among these individuals is very important and must be maintained at all times.

Although each project equipment manager is responsible for his or her individual projects, the project equipment managers also spend a considerable amount of time keeping abreast of developments in their respective areas of expertise. The department has representatives at all major equipment shows throughout the country, such as those sponsored by the Radiological Society of North America and the American Society of Medical Technologists.

> **With the project equipment manager as a one-point contact, all problems involved with equipment for the project can be quickly addressed.**

This allows project equipment managers to constantly update the equipment list produced by the computer so that all spaces are equipped with state-of-the-art items.

Of major importance to this type of computer system is the consistency of communication with the hospitals, which has proven to be extremely valuable when these hospitals encounter construction problems. With the project equipment manager as a one-point contact, all problems involved with equipment for the project can be quickly addressed.

Technical advisory boards

To provide the most effective equipment list possible, HCA has established technical advisory boards for the areas of respiratory therapy, nursing service, laboratory, radiology, dietetics, physical therapy, pharmacy and materiel management. Meeting with board members twice each year for three days and being in constant telephone contact with them provides HCA with information regarding every item on the equipment list.

Technical advisory board members are selected from hospitals of every size and from every area of the country. Members serve for two years, which allows them to become accustomed to the construction process and to become acquainted with all of the methods used. The value of these people cannot be overemphasized. Not only have they provided considerable expertise to the construction and renovation projects, but they have also served as consultants throughout the corporation.

During the three-day programs scheduled for the technical advisory boards, vendors are often invited to demonstrate their products and educational programs have also been instituted in some areas of management. This allows the board members to be involved in the evaluation of new products and methods and to be more effective in their hospital positions. Each year people have been increasingly interested in serving on the boards, and this is encouraged. With the continued growth of the corporation, this pool of talent has been an invaluable asset and HCA continues to draw from this pool to maintain the three-day technical advisory program at the highest level possible.

Order of business

The initiation of a new construction project within HCA begins with a feasibility study by the Design and Development Department. The equipment section of the Materiel Management Department is notified of this new project by what is called a zebra sheet. This sheet lists those departments and spaces within the department that are to be included for a new hospital or for additions or renovations within an existing facility.

Using this report and a written program prepared by the Programming Department, the project equipment manager compares each of these with schematic drawings obtained from the architect to produce the first proposed budget. This budget is reviewed within the Materiel Management Department then submitted to the Certificate of Need Department for review and evaluation. The project equipment manager is often asked to testify at health services administration (HSA) hearings or to present this list to physicians, hospital personnel or other appropriate people.

Once the certificate of need has been issued, the project equipment manager takes the list to the hospital and meets with each department head and other appropriate personnel, including physicians, to review the equipment. At this time, changes can be made, if necessary, and the project equipment manager can establish a strong communication link with all people involved in the project. This initial visit requires approximately three days for each project; however, this time is well spent as the knowledge gained and rapport established will be extremely valuable during the project.

After reviewing the project with all appropriate hospital personnel, the project equipment manager re-inputs into the computer each individual space and item

within that space, reflecting those changes made during the hospital meetings. From this input, a reviewed and approved budget is produced. This list is again taken to the hospital and reviewed with the same personnel. The list has been in use for more than four years, and few changes have been required in the reviewed and approved budget.

After the second review with hospital personnel, the budget is locked into the computer, which has been programmed to produce the purchase orders for every item in time to ensure proper delivery. By handling the project in this manner, many items can be purchased, such as dietary equipment, surgical lights and sterilizers, that often are included in the contractor's budget by non-HCA hospitals. The delivery schedule and purchase orders must be constantly monitored. With this computerized method, each project equipment manager can manage approximately 18 projects. With a manual method, a project equipment manager could manage only about 6 projects.

All purchase orders are prepared by the computer, and all items are arranged by date of order, to ensure proper delivery. All order dates are based on the opening date or completion date of the project. The computer has produced a far more accurate purchase order system than could have been achieved with manual methods. On a quarterly basis, each vendor is sent a list of all items in the computer from their company. The vendor reviews the list and makes appropriate changes on dates of orders, dates of delivery and prices.

Many purchase orders are issued as far as one year in advance of completion. These are for sterilizers, surgical lights and other items that are owner furnished and contractor installed. If the vendor delivers these items at the appropriate time, on-site storage, which is often difficult to find, is not necessary.

The computer also produces a receiving report, which is sent to the project manager and can be used by the hospital personnel to notify HCA of the delivery of the item. When a purchase order is mailed to the vendor, it is stamped with a request that the vendor acknowledge the order within ten days so that HCA will know if the vendor can meet the delivery date and the specifications set forth on the purchase order. A log showing each purchase order is checked every 30 days until the item is received. This procedure has been extremely important in identifying problems at an early stage of the project, rather than at the time of delivery when it is too late to solve the problem.

The receiving function

Of major importance in the process is the individual in charge of receiving equipment at the project site. This person must be aware of all items received and know all proper procedures for filing damage claims and other appropriate paperwork so that immediate changes can be made if a problem does exist. Without exception, there is a great deal of activity in the first 60 days of a project, when the budget is being finalized and all items are being selected. The next and most important activities will begin approximately 30 days from completion of the project when the majority of the equipment items, such as furniture, will begin to arrive on the site. This has to be coordinated very closely with the general contractor to ensure that all items reach the proper space.

Inspection visits

The project equipment manager schedules trips to the project site at appropriate intervals during construction to ensure that all information is properly communicated. It is very important that the manager visit the project approximately three weeks before completion to walk through the project and examine every piece of equipment. Too many times equipment is installed in the wrong space, such as an examining table being placed in an emergency room instead of close to the nursing station.

This final walk-through saves the project equipment manager time by eliminating many of the problems experienced at this particular phase of construction. If the visit to the project is not made at least three weeks before opening and a problem is discovered, there is no time to solve the problem and to have a new piece of equipment sent to the project. If the visit is made before arrival of all equipment, then problems cannot be properly identified.

Vendor input

During this last visit, many of the training programs and in-service education programs can be instituted and arranged by the project equipment manager working with the vendors. This can be extremely important if the department head and the individuals using the new equipment have not been properly trained or are new employees. Most vendors have excellent in-service education programs and will work closely with hospital personnel to use these programs to the best advantage. In most cases, if a vendor will train two people, it is best to allow one person to go through the school first, and to send the second person approximately 90 days later, after the equipment has been used.

Often questions and problems can be more properly addressed after the equipment has been in place for some time. No matter how much time is spent in planning, unforeseen situations always arise in the last few days before opening. These problems must be handled as they arise and cannot always be anticipated.

Throughout a project, all communication with vendors, quotations and proposals are handled by the project equipment manager through the corporate office. This allows the project equipment manager to be in control of all discussions through the project. It is not uncommon to have problems when local representatives of vendors present themselves to a department head and arrive at decisions that will not fit into the program for that particular facility. The input of individuals at the projects is not discouraged; however, changes after the budget has been finalized can cause many problems. To minimize these problems, HCA asks each contract vendor to appoint one representative to handle all HCA purchase orders. This allows HCA to communicate with one individual and eliminates having to keep up with all regional and district offices throughout the country.

Obviously, this can be an advantage from a price standpoint, since the individuals who work with HCA are aware of all purchase orders and not just those in any one area. However, this policy can at times cause considerable confusion among the vendors until they realize the importance of early specifications. By the time a local representative sees a project underway, all equipment and construction specifications for that project have been completed. Changes in specifications during the con-

struction period may be allowed if equipment is introduced to the market that changes the state of the art and offers a great advantage to the hospital. Again, proper planning from the beginning of the project is the key to ensuring that changes are not made at a later date.

Cut sheets

Perhaps one of the greatest problems faced during any construction project is providing the architects with complete specifications of all equipment to be furnished. This is particularly true of those items that are owner furnished and contractor installed, such as surgical lights, sterilizers and television sets. It is sometimes forgotten that architects must be provided with information on equipment that needs special wiring, such as Coulter counters, ultrasound units and other sophisticated equipment.

Many vendors are unaware of what an architect or contractor means by a "cut sheet." Vendors tend to provide information sheets that give the type of procedures equipment will perform but that lack the necessary information that engineers and architects must be aware of early in a project, such as amperage, voltage, size and weight.

Such information is provided by HCA to architects and contractors in an equipment brochure prepared for each project. This brochure contains not only necessary information, but photographs of all equipment to be installed by the contractor, with notes on special wiring, air conditioning or other requirements related to architectural design. When the brochure is prepared, a meeting is held with the contractor and project architect to review and to place each item of equipment on the plan so that everyone is aware of all specifications. Changes can be made at this time if they are necessary. Changes made after final drawings have been produced are very costly and must be avoided if possible.

Since most hospital personnel are involved in a construction project only once or twice, it is the project manager who must constantly review all items. The important factor is to identify all items at the beginning of the project, to be sure that the scope of the project is very clearly defined and that changes in equipment and ensuing construction changes are held to an absolute minimum. Although this sounds somewhat simplistic, it is very difficult to achieve when specifications are developed two years in advance of a completed project.

ACQUISITIONS IN AN OPERATING FACILITY

As was pointed out, the HCA philosophy of decentralization and local autonomy lends itself to a capital equipment acquisition procedure that is similar to that of a stand-alone hospital—one that does not belong to an investor-owned corporation.

An HCA-owned hospital that wishes to buy additional or replacement equipment develops a capital equipment budget in July and August of each year. Each hospital submits its budget to its division vice president for review and approval.

The division vice president sends the capital budgets submitted by each hospital to corporate materiel management for review and comment as to manufacturer, model and price. Corporate materiel management does not approve or disapprove these budgets but serves as an advisor and consultant for the division vice president.

All hospitals are aware of this procedure, and most administrators contact the corporate materiel management staff for review of and comment on their planned budget requests. Most hospitals are aware of the corporate materiel management department's computerized equipment list and request printouts for spaces or departments that they are planning to equip.

In preparation for capital equipment acquisition, a hospital should:

1. Make sure that there is a real need for the piece of equipment.
2. Communicate with all personnel who may be affected, such as the department who requested it; the engineering department, to ensure that sufficient space, electrical requirements, heating and air conditioning, and ventilation are provided if needed; and materiel management, to ensure proper purchase orders and receiving procedures.
3. Make sure that the vendor can provide in-service education and proper service.

The capital equipment purchasing policies of a multihospital organization must reflect the philosophy of that organization. If that philosophy represents a centralized, controlled environment, then the purchasing policies must reflect this. If the philosophy gives autonomy to each facility and emphasizes a decentralized concept, then the purchasing policies must follow this concept.

In either case, the policy must be designed to create an environment conducive to the establishment of an effective, economical and creatively productive facility that reflects an appropriate program for the present and the future.

Group purchasing—the great debate

David M. Baker
Director
Materiel Management
St. John's Mercy Medical Center
St. Louis, Missouri

WHILE DEBATE still rages on the benefits and disadvantages of hospital group purchasing, it is the undeniable growth of the groups that makes the strongest case for their success. Still, the recent General Accounting Office (GAO) report, *Study of Purchasing and Materials Management Functions in Private Hospitals,* raises questions about the real effectiveness of groups: "Hospitals should consider whether group purchasing saves them money. Comparing prices for similar items purchased by the four hospitals [studied] shows that while some were obtained at lower prices through group agreements than independently, for others the opposite was true."[1]

This debate is now the hospital's challenge. Hospitals must survey their group efforts, assess them, and act to maximize purchasing power. The relatively short history of hospital group purchasing and the rapid growth of the numbers of groups and their contracts present a body of experiences that is adequately broad yet of manageable size for evaluation.

THE DEVELOPMENT OF PURCHASING GROUPS

The early stage

Before looking at all groups today, it is important to note what the birth of groups accomplished. The early group offered voluntary participation and required much coaxing and cajoling of member purchasing people. Early group efforts resulted in a "membership drive" that gradually garnered enough support to do at least one critical thing—establish a price frame of reference or a price ceiling for a product throughout the area served. Because all hospitals were for the first time privy to more pricing knowledge, "bad deals" were exposed and usually corrected. Solution contracts have been the single most successful target of group purchasing, and few hospitals remain that receive only a 30 percent discount on solutions. This ceiling effect exists everywhere a group exists, but its benefits are hard to measure. Those most critical of groups often overlook this basic fact. Many existing group efforts are still in this early stage, while others have progressed to the next step.

Second stage

Looking further at types of groups reveals a second stage. A group at this level, still with voluntary member participation, has experienced two phenomena: (1) an established camaraderie among members, and (2) contract atrophy. After ceilings were established with mediocre participation from the group (whose members are now starting to like each other), stagnation of group impact or contract atrophy occurs. Contract atrophy is a symptom of any group still at this stage. Usually members here begin to recognize the need to overcome this impotence. This revelation brings most groups to the "committed volume" stage.

Committed volume stage

Most of the recent literature in group purchasing lauds the impact of committed volume as opposed to the earlier form of voluntary group purchasing. A survey of benefits need not be restated here, but let it suffice to say that whenever one guarantees a conversion to a product or the purchase of a certain volume, anyone selling that product will respond with better pricing. Reducing the uncertainty for vendors reduces their risk and enables them to shave their margins.

It should be noted, however, that committed volume can take many forms. The Hospital Association of Metropolitan St. Louis (HAMSTL) is a voluntary group by program, but at any given time, when its advisory committee so decides, it can advertise which and how many hospitals choose to precommit on a particular contract before bids go out. This approach has shown progress in several areas. Gary Wittrock, the purchasing director of the St. Louis group, explains, "The success of a committed effort is not necessarily contingent upon 100 percent involvement of membership. But a predetermined commitment—even if it is only one-half the members—still achieves desired results." While total strict committed volume will achieve the lowest prices, hospitals should not be blinded to the benefits of limited committed volume such as that used by HAMSTL. Mr. Wittrock continues, "This dualism allows a blending of two methodologies which provides both cost containment and that measure of flexibility needed by many members."[2]

This flexibility, while sometimes acquired at the expense of the very "best" price, allows hospitals to avoid the trauma and cost of product conversions. Nevertheless, any group at this stage can find success in containing some costs. The partial commitment is sufficient to overcome the contract atrophy of the earlier stage.

GROUP PURCHASING OF EQUIPMENT

More groups are now venturing into the equipment arena for contracts. This is due partly to the fact that many of the supply areas are saturated by group contracts, but also because equipment manufacturers have taken note of the group movement and responded with increasingly generous discounts. The Mercy Province of St. Louis, for instance, has generated great savings in equipment purchases through its contracts with AMSCO, Everest & Jennings, and more recently even Hewlett Packard, although the discount in the latter case is relatively small. These contracts have great potential because of the increasing number of hospitals now involved in building programs and expansion of diagnostic services.

The Sisters of the Third Order of St. Francis, in Peoria, Illinois, concentrates heavily in the equipment arena and has many of the same contracts as the Mercy group. In fact, since this purchasing group now markets its contract to hospitals nationwide, its greatest and most immediate value to any prospective member is that, faced with an impending purchase from AMSCO, for instance, simply signing up with the group affords the hospital an instant 10 or 15 percent discount.

While the rush to grab available equipment discounts is on and must be used to advantage by all hospitals whenever possible, a future consideration cannot be ignored. Might equipment distributors simply inflate their list prices and offer discounts to give the appearance of submitting to the power of groups, while in fact their net prices and margins remain the same? Time will tell. A far less jaundiced view would consider that there is, in fact, much for the equipment manufacturers to gain through group purchasing contracts, including greater ease of closing a sale, and enhanced ability to "get a foot in the door" when needed. There is evidence that equipment selections have certainly been influenced by existing hospital contracts.

A CHOICE OF GROUPS

As if struggling with group participation were not enough, hospitals must now face another dilemma brought on by the proliferation of groups. Often the question is no longer how to use group purchasing, but which group to use. More and more groups have appeared because of geography, religious order affiliation, or other considerations. Inevitably, overlapping has

*Since some purchasing groups are so-
liciting membership throughout the
country for usage of their contracts
based on fees, every hospital is a customer and can shop for the group
that best serves its needs.*

occurred. For St. John's Mercy Medical
Center in St. Louis, there is one group
buying effort by the Sisters of Mercy
within its province and one by the local
hospital association (HAMSTL). The
groups, in effect, often compete with each
other. The position of the hospital has
been to select the better of the two
contracts when faced with this dilemma,
but even then many problems remained.

Many hospitals have recently found
themselves in similar quandaries. Since
some purchasing groups are soliciting
membership throughout the country for
usage of their contracts based on fees,
every hospital in the country is now a
customer and can shop for the group that
best serves its needs. The pressure is on the
hospital to be prudent. Jewish Hospital in
St. Louis, a member of the Consortium of
Jewish Hospitals (CJH) and HAMSTL,
deals with this problem very simply. Its
materiels management director, Jim
Schmitz, explains, "Because both of our
groups are voluntary, we are free to select
that contract that best serves our hospital."[3]

However, Mr. Schmitz also points out
that groups do not necessarily compete all
the time. In fact, a national group such as
CJH, with members throughout the country, can complement a more localized,
geographically centered effort such as the
St. Louis organization. He continues,
"Many supply items do not lend themselves to a nationwide effort. Examples
would include office supplies and linen
services, where the local effort is the only
practical choice."[4]

PROBLEMS FACED BY GROUPS

Director competence

Regardless of which group a hospital
joins, or which strategies a group employs,
little will be accomplished without the
efforts of a good group coordinator. This
"salesperson" must help foster cooperation through rapport and involvement of
hospital purchasing group members. If a
member disapproves of the methods used
or has no input into the contracting
process, its participation might well be
expected to be poor. Some group directors, while excellent at the mechanics of
bidding and negotiating, do not sell their
product effectively. This is of critical
importance to any voluntary effort. It is
the group director who must shoulder the
burden of group purchasing's several
common dilemmas, not the least of which
is participation.

Fairness

A second major dilemma of group
purchasing involves fairness. A group must
maintain good information and be very
thorough to display good purchasing
mechanics. Good mechanics will in turn
help the group in its struggle to be fair to
vendors and member hospitals. Examples
of poor mechanics would include:

• Omission of a vendor from a bid list;

- Use of inaccurate "spread sheets" to review bids;
- Lack of hospital usage figures; and
- Sloppy dissemination of information.

It should be noted, however, that in every bidding process there can be only one winner. Disgruntled vendors will be a fact of life, regardless of the efforts made. Moreover, these vendors will be quick to plead their cases.

Direction

Thirdly, the purchasing group must channel its energy to areas offering the greatest rewards. Many groups have found that contracts with manufacturers offer more than those with distributors or dealers.

The Sisters of the Third Order of St. Francis has embraced this approach and has been very successful by concentrating on manufacturers. Because 80 percent or more of the final price paid by the hospital goes to the manufacturer, it is logical that the greater potential cost concession should come from the manufacturer rather than the dealer.

The Order employs a unique tactic that shows great promise for other groups. A supply contract with a manufacturer may be serviced by different dealers or a dealer of the hospital's choosing. This separation of the purchase and service responsibilities eliminates many problems for members and encourages participation.

One price for all members?

Another problem facing groups is the "single price dilemma." For a vendor to give a group one price means it has to submit that price for the 100-bed hospital 150 miles from its warehouse, and the 1,000-bed hospital nearby. While debate still rages in many circles, some groups have come to realize that this is unrealistic and that, in fact, contracts should be tiered or have some built-in incentives to enlist the participation of the 1,000-bed hospital while not overly penalizing the 100-bed hospital. The fact is, purchasing in quantity allows for better pricing. Although this seems logical, much anger may exist over this issue within a group's membership. If groups do not recognize this problem and modify their contracts to accommodate their large and small members, they will eventually alienate their larger members who will constantly be solicited by vendors with deals and offers that they cannot ignore. Smaller hospitals should not resent larger hospitals for this "special treatment" because in the long term it will mean progress for the group as a whole.

ASSESSMENT OF PURCHASING GROUPS

These problems and others have done little to slow the growth of groups, but much to spark debate on their effectiveness. One reason for the continuing debate is that the benefits of groups are not easily quantifiable. Dollar savings reports are rough estimates at best, and larger hospitals are often tempted to assume that they could do better alone—although that judgment is purely subjective.

In another recent study commissioned by the U.S. Senate Subcommittee on Health, the GAO concludes that "membership in group purchasing did not necessarily result in hospitals achieving the lowest price available in the area."[5] Although this statement implies group ineffectiveness, that should not be inferred. Not having the lowest price in town does not mean the group has not lowered costs. In fact, the lowest price in town could be a result of the group's "ceiling effect" mentioned earlier.

But aside from price, there are many other less tangible benefits of group membership, including the sharing of ideas and information. The knowledge and professional development generated are critical to anyone in hospital purchasing today. Increased group effort can provide purchasing professionals with another advantage that is sometimes overlooked. That is *time*. Buying through good group contracts can save time and allow more attention to the management of materiel, which sometimes gets less attention than it deserves.

As hospitals realize the potential cost savings in controlling supplies, inventory, and usage, more efforts will be directed there. Group purchasing will allow many purchasing professionals to make the transition to materiel management. If materiel management is to grow as a science, group purchasing may well be a major reason for this growth. This partnership of two efforts offers the greatest promise for hospital cost containment in the 1980s.

REFERENCES

1. General Accounting Office. *Study of Purchasing and Materials Management Functions in Private Hospitals*, Volume 1, PSAD-79-58A (Washington, D.C.: Government Printing Office April 1979).
2. Wittrock, G., Personal Communication, September 1980.
3. Schmitz, J., Personal Communication, September 1980.
4. Ibid.
5. General Accounting Office. *Study of Purchasing and Materials Management Functions in Private Hospitals.*

Overcoming barriers to group purchasing

Charles E. Housley
Associate Administrator
Saint Anthony Hospital
Columbus, Ohio

IN THESE TIMES of cost consciousness and cost containment, group purchasing has gained much support from hospital administrators and regulators. Many hospitals use group purchasing to some extent, but in the average hospital it represents only about 10 percent of the total volume of purchases. Certainly group purchasing can be more widely utilized. If group purchasing is an answer to cost containment, why do not hospitals use group purchasing more?

COMMON BARRIERS TO GROUP PURCHASING

Barriers to group purchasing can be erected by the hospital, group purchasing organization or vendor. Gaining an understanding of the barriers is the first step toward dismantling them.

Lack of commitment from agents and vendors

One often hears from the vendors and hospital administrators that a solution to group purchasing problems is group commitment, but group purchasing must go far beyond mere commitment. Commitment is meaningless unless that commitment carries a real obligation. Purchasing agents should be obligated to participate in group purchasing, and the group should be obligated to obtain better prices and services for its members.

However, it seems that group purchasing has not matured to this point yet. Group purchasing is still in its infancy, and in many cases it only means that a group of hospitals have indicated that they would be willing to participate in group purchasing. This is far from an obligation. To induce hospitals to obligate their purchasing agents to use group purchasing the group would have to guarantee results immediately, in the near future and in the long run.

Another factor to consider is the attitude of the vendor. As the hospitals lack a sense of commitment and obligation, the vendors do also. The vendors give lip service to group purchasing, but their prices tend to reflect individual pricing rather than group pricing. For instance, if the vendor's catalog indicates an individual price and one or two volume prices, then the vendor who has a definite commitment and obligation to group purchasing should also indicate a price category for group purchasing. The vendor may have some items that are not subject to the group purchasing price, and these would be excluded from that category. For the rest of the items, the vendor should indicate pricing levels for group purchasing.

For example, the vendor may have a price of $5 for a particular item purchased in quantities up to 6; 6 to 25 may cost $4.75 each, and over 25, $4.60. This is normal pricing for most catalogs and indicates that volume produces better prices. If a vendor is really committed to group purchasing, the pricing should list such categories as: group price for 1,000 to 5,000 beds, $4.50; 5,000 to 10,000 beds, $4.40; 10,000 to 20,000 beds, $4.30; over 20,000 beds, $4.25.

One cannot guarantee under the traditional rules of group purchasing that there will be a definite volume. Therefore, to induce the vendor to undertake an obligation (not just a commitment) each hospital in the group purchasing effort must be obligated to committed dollar volume in the group purchasing efforts. The vendor may want to establish group purchasing prices based on dollar volume per bed; for example, for group purchasing of 5,000 to 10,000 beds a vendor may state, "Each hospital would get this price with a committed volume of at least $1,000 per bed per item." This is what it will take in the future to make group purchasing worthwhile and credible.

Lack of credibility in group purchasing

The typical purchasing agent still has little faith in group purchasing, and group purchasing directors have doubts about agents who make up the group. They feel that the agents will undermine group purchasing if they get an opportunity to make a better deal individually.

Some vendors come up with makeshift prices and then complain that the hospitals do not give them their business even under group purchasing arrangements. This vicious circle must be broken once and for all. If group purchasing is good for the hospital, then the hospital should be willing to be obligated. If the hospitals are really obligated to group purchasing then it will be good for the vendors, and the vendors will promote group purchasing in their pricing and marketing strategies.

One of the problems with group purchasing is the lack of evidence that it will work better than any other form of purchasing. Until this has been clearly demonstrated it will be difficult for the agent, group purchasing director and vendor to have total faith in the group purchasing concept.

A threat to the hospital purchasing agent

Many hospital purchasing agents feel that group purchasing detracts from their power and authority. After the purchasing group has negotiated a price and before the purchasing agents have agreed to it, many of the agents feel an obligation to talk to the vendors to see if they can get a better price individually. This undermines the group purchasing effort. It would appear that every group purchasing endeavor has one or more agents who seem to be more loyal to the vendor than to the group. Many vendors will take advantage of this situation, and as long as there are agents who undermine the group, there will be vendors who will lower prices to keep group purchasing from succeeding.

Today's purchasing agent should be more interested in getting the best possible price and providing evidence of this price than in keeping up contacts with specific sales representatives. Friendship and favors

should end as the sales representative comes into the hospital. The agent should look at price and service and negotiate accordingly. Quality is not an issue here because the quality control of most reputable companies is ensured by the various regulatory and monitoring entities.

Agents should make group purchasing work in their favor, and with the various tools of purchasing such as individual purchase power, group purchasing, prime vending and stockless purchasing, the agent should be able to ascertain very quickly what would be in the best interests of the hospital. There are ways to determine the best price although vendors today make it very difficult to find the best price among the various vendors. Many vendors who are selling and marketing the same type of item will have a different price structure for different aspects of that supply category. For instance, intravenous (I.V.) solutions may have three different prices: one for intravenous solutions, one for administration sets and one for nutritional products.

The only sure way for the purchasing agent to tell which offer is the best for the hospital is to calculate the cost of each line item by the volume that the hospital uses and the price each vendor has quoted. The purchasing agent may have to perform this calculation on 50 to 150 line items before the end result is apparent. However, the results will be clear-cut even to the inexperienced eye.

The purchasing agent of today should not be threatened by group purchasing, but agents who do not take into serious consideration the possibilities and advantages for their hospitals are actually threatening their own positions. The calculations mentioned above should be kept on record by the prudent agent, and should be shared with the purchasing group director and the hospital administrator. If more and more agents would use this type of projection and forecasting, then the vendors would be more straightforward in providing good prices for the hospitals.

Getting the best price is the responsibility of every purchasing agent. Whether this is done through individual buying, group purchasing or prime vending has a lot to do with the obligation of the hospital and the portrayal of this obligation to the vendor. If anyone is to feel threatened in this situation, it should be the vendor who does not recognize the determination of the hospital and offer the best possible price.

Lack of effectiveness on the part of group purchasing directors

Many group purchasing directors would say that unsuccessful group bidders will undercut the groups' prices to obtain or retain a hospital's business. A hospital may obtain short-term gains by purchasing from a nongroup vendor, but the practice can detract from long-range group effectiveness.

If a vendor is willing to undercut to get one hospital's business, why does not that vendor give the lowest price to the entire group and get the total group's business? The mystery still remains: How can a hospital of 200 to 300 beds get a better price than a group representing 5,000 to 10,000 beds? Could it be that the group price is just not that good? Could it be that the vendor the hospitals have chosen really did not offer the best possible price?

A commitment to group purchasing cannot be fulfilled by the hospitals alone. This commitment of trust must be among three parties—the hospital, group purchasing organization and vendor. All three play a very important role. If there is sufficient commitment and communication, then it will be extremely difficult to have a vendor retain a hospital's business by underbidding the group.

One of the most comprehensive studies on hospitals and the prices they pay for various items has been conducted by the General Accounting Office (GAO). In the study, they define a group purchasing association as an organization composed of hospitals of different sizes that have banded together to realize cost savings through purchasing in larger quantities. The contention is that a group, because of its greater negotiating power, can obtain better discounts than the members can get individually.

However, surveys on which the report was based show that group associations

---

Surveys show that group associations did not necessarily pay the lowest prices in the area, and some even had the highest prices for the area.

---

did not necessarily pay the lowest prices in the area, and some even had the highest prices for the area. Cities where this occurred include Columbus, Cincinnati, Miami, Atlanta and Seattle. Group purchasing directors reported that some bidders who had not been awarded the contract would undercut the group price to get an individual hospital's business, and one hospital reported that it had used the group's price to negotiate the same price from another vendor. Furthermore, some hospitals yield to the pressure of personnel and medical staff preferences when making decisions on purchasing.

Vendors fear loss of profits

One may ask, "Why should hospitals buying in groups get better prices?" In almost all group purchasing situations, individual hospitals order, receive and reorder merchandise from a selected vendor. The selected vendor may have been getting all of that hospital's business from the beginning. Since hospitals in most purchasing groups do not buy in volumes of 6 or 12 months (because it would not be practical for them to do so), and since many group purchasing associations do not have their own warehouses, where do the savings come from? Where can the vendor really save or reduce costs in order to pass the savings along to the hospital? No group purchasing study that I have seen has shown that the vendor's bottom line has actually been negatively affected because of group purchasing. In fact, there is some indication that vendors just redistribute their prices and still come out with the same bottom line, shifting costs to other hospitals not in purchasing groups.

For group purchasing to be effective and to have credibility among all the hospitals and purchasing agents, some of these problems must be resolved. From the standpoint of the hospital and the hospital purchasing agent, group purchasing must and should produce low prices— better than a purchasing agent can get from any other source. From the stand-

point of the vendor, those hospitals in the group must be not only committed but obligated to purchase the volumes that have been predetermined. However, many groups do not commit to any set volume. This also detracts from the credibility of group purchasing. So the terms from the vendor's point of view of group purchasing must be clearly stated in writing. They must give prices based on volume, and they must indicate committed volumes based on the hospital's needs over a specified period of time.

Failure to share pricing information

One of the things that would help bring about a clearer understanding of group purchasing would be the sharing of price information by all the hospitals in any area. The purchasing agents should be aware of what everyone else is paying and under what conditions they are purchasing.

Again, the GAO study showed that many purchasing agents are unaware of what other hospitals pay. The impression surveyors received was that agents generally did not share price information. One of the reasons suggested was that if they find they are paying higher prices, they could lose their jobs! Another reason was that the vendors had told them not to tell their prices.

The study revealed that hospital administrators also did not know how the prices they were paying compared with those paid by other hospitals, and some expressed a need for some system to share information on supply costs. Knowledge of customary prices could lead to lower prices: the reasoning is that equal knowledge of all parties helps protect against favoritism and profiteering. The hospitals

Medical-Surgical Profile

1. Foley Cath Tray

Sterile plastic tray with: closed system 2000cc drainage bag; 2-way, 16fr, 5 cc silicone foley catheter; 1 oz povidone-iodine solution; safety pin and rubber band; tube clip; 2 vinyl exam gloves; drape; underpad, 5 gram lubricant; 5 rayon balls; 10cc syringe with 9 cc sterile water.

Unit Ea. Tray

		Region 1			Region 2			Region 3			Region 4			Region 5		
		L	M	H	L	M	H	L	M	H	L	M	H	L	M	H
BED SIZE	1-249	8.08	8.76	10.20	ID	ID	ID	7.55	8.69	9.92	4.73	8.63	11.37	6.41	6.64	13.89
	250-Over	5.99	6.62	7.25	6.67	9.05	12.42	5.08	7.91	.62	4.99	7.54	11.32	5.08	8.58	9.95
METHOD OF PURCHASE	Individual	5.99	7.25	8.55	6.67	8.15	12.42	7.13	8.05	8.97	4.73	9.19	11.37	5.08	8.88	13.89
	Group	8.76	9.83	10.20	9.95	10.10	10.26	7.20	8.51	9.92	5.99	7.25	8.93	6.22	7.52	9.77
	Prime Vendor	ID	ID	ID	ID	ID	ID	5.08	8.47	9.36	7.43	8.71	10.06	ID	ID	ID

		Region 6			Region 7			Region 8			Region 9			National		
		L	M	H	L	M	H	L	M	H	L	M	H	L	M	H
BED SIZE	1-249	6.14	7.38	12.17	7.47	9.24	10.27	7.18	7.69	10.54	5.16	7.92	10.95	4.73	8.49	13.89
	250-Over	5.80	6.84	8.47	6.10	8.32	12.08	7.37	8.64	9.92	6.67	10.69	12.20	4.99	8.01	12.42
METHOD OF PURCHASE	Individual	5.80	8.38	12.17	6.10	7.22	11.13	7.18	7.27	7.37	8.45	10.58	10.95	4.73	8.35	13.89
	Group	6.07	7.03	9.79	7.52	8.50	12.08	9.92	10.23	10.54	6.22	7.58	11.62	5.99	7.62	12.08
	Prime Vendor	6.14	6.84	9.02	7.47	10.05	10.27	7.24	7.69	8.15	5.16	10.69	12.20	5.08	8.47	12.20

2. Catheter, Solution Basin, and Glove Kit

Sterile solution container, 14-16fr. whistle tip w/thumb control rubber or plastic catheter, vinyl glove

Unit Ea. Kit

		Region 1			Region 2			Region 3			Region 4			Region 5		
		L	M	H	L	M	H	L	M	H	L	M	H	L	M	H
BED SIZE	1-249	0.79	0.95	1.12	0.61	1.46	1.89	0.50	0.53	1.26	0.50	0.64	1.19	0.55	0.56	0.57
	250-Over	0.54	0.65	0.76	0.44	0.56	0.62	0.49	0.60	1.88	0.41	0.51	0.64	0.43	0.65	1.53
METHOD OF PURCHASE	Individual	0.54	0.79	1.12	0.54	0.58	0.62	0.49	0.55	0.89	0.41	0.50	1.19	0.43	0.63	0.88
	Group	ID	ID	ID	0.44	1.46	1.89	0.52	0.56	0.60	0.56	0.63	0.64	0.50	0.60	1.53
	Prime Vendor	ID	ID	ID	ID	ID	ID	0.50	0.93	1.88	0.63	0.64	0.66	ID	ID	ID

		Region 6			Region 7			Region 8			Region 9			National		
		L	M	H	L	M	H	L	M	H	L	M	H	L	M	H
BED SIZE	1-249	0.46	0.84	2.40	0.56	0.58	0.60	0.52	0.75	0.79	0.61	0.73	1.19	0.46	0.73	2.40
	250-Over	0.40	0.63	0.82	0.40	0.72	1.77	0.62	0.64	0.68	0.55	0.80	0.93	0.40	0.61	1.88
METHOD OF PURCHASE	Individual	0.40	0.80	1.49	0.40	0.66	1.77	0.62	0.64	0.67	0.55	0.73	0.87	0.40	0.62	1.77
	Group	0.46	0.79	1.46	ID	ID	ID	0.62	0.68	0.75	0.65	0.92	1.19	0.44	0.63	1.89
	Prime Vendor	ID	ID	ID	0.56	0.71	1.30	0.62	0.65	0.79	0.77	0.85	0.93	0.50	0.74	2.40

September 1981 · No. 2

Figure 1. Comparison of prices paid for supplies by hospitals and purchasing groups.

can also learn how the suppliers bid on hospital requirements. If hospitals begin by sharing price information on the most basic supply needs, they can go on from there to share experiences on value analysis and standardization and expand their knowledge considerably.

It is true that agents do not compare prices. There are many reasons for this, none of which is well founded. In the September 1981 edition of the *Aspen Hospital Purchasing Price Index,*[1] it can be seen that hospitals pay different prices, and in many cases smaller hospitals get better prices. (See Figure 1.) As long as hospitals continue to pay more through groups than they do individually, they will be open to criticism. The effective group purchasing association should know the prices paid and should start at this point to negotiate for better prices. In other words, well-informed group purchasing directors will know what prices are being paid for all items in several different areas and will use this information in skilled negotiations to obtain a good price for their individual group associations. In the future the negotiation of prices will be the primary purpose of the group purchasing association.

Lack of leadership

Leadership must come from all parties. It is hard to be optimistic and enthusiastic about a concept in which you do not believe. Therefore, it is necessary to have an agent who is supportive of group purchasing in actions as well as words. Many traditional agents have not supported group purchasing and indeed still tend to oppose group purchasing.

However, good leadership principles stress that the agent should get behind the group purchasing efforts. Instead of dividing the group, the agent should help bring the group together. Some modern agents tend to be more supportive of group purchasing; however, their prices do not always speak well for their efforts.

There are certain characteristics that indicate leadership ability in the agent. Most important is a desire to get the best possible prices for the institution. Pride in one's own hospital can be made evident without compromising commitment to the group. Second, a leader must be well informed. Agents must know the prices that are being paid in the area and seek to better those prices through the best possible ethical means. Third, the agent should have a participative spirit. The agent should say, "What's best for the group is best for my hospital," and should seek to get the best prices and service through group efforts. Pride in the group effort is a characteristic of good leadership. When the group efforts are beneficial to the hospital's goal, then the agent can take pride in the hospital's participation in the group. Finally, the agent should show the leadership trait of endurance. He or she should not stop until the best possible group effort has been achieved.

The most important leadership quality in a group purchasing director is initiative. The director must have a goal for the group and a plan for attaining the goal. This goal must be communicated to all members of the group. The director must be able to deal with different individuals with different ideas and mold them into a team to get the best prices.

The leadership of group purchasing is

often misunderstood by the agents. The agents tend to think that the director is trying to outperform them and to make them look bad to their administrators. Many agents do not feel that their administrators give them enough time; therefore, they are jealous of the time that administrators spend with the group director. Agents may feel that the director is keeping something from them and communicating it to the administrators rather than to them. Directors must be able to reassure the agents that group purchasing will make all parties look good and no one look bad.

The director must be assertive and able to set goals and objectives for the vendors to meet. The director must be able to take the ideas of the agents, put them into a group objective and get better results from the vendors than the agents could ever get individually. The director is really an agent of the hospital purchasing agent and an extension of the efforts of that agent.

A team effort on the part of all agents and the director making up the group is needed. Together they must present an unwavering front to gain the respect of the vendors. Credibility is essential for the director, both from the perspective of the agent and the vendor. Many a group has failed because of the lack of leadership. The director must be able to show results to the agents and administrators and to Blue Cross and other third party regulators. These results have to be clear-cut and demonstrable in dollars and cents.

Conflicts that arise between hospitals and vendors

Do most vendors want to participate in group purchasing? Most successful companies that sell medical-surgical supplies to hospitals will indicate that they have to make a certain percentage in profits to stay in business. Many of them will point out several companies that have used loss leaders and cut prices so much that today they are out of business. These companies would argue that it has not helped the hospital industry, and certainly not the hospitals, to have a supplier go bankrupt or out of business.

If the agent or director never mentioned group purchasing to a sales representative, would there ever be mention of group purchasing? Probably not. Common sense indicates that if group purchasing is effective, then the hospital vendor will be making less profit. Then why would a vendor ever want to enter into a group purchasing contract? The most likely answer is that the vendor must compete with other companies who are participating in group purchasing endeavors.

Today the successful company will have several options for a hospital, namely, good individual prices, group purchasing prices, prime vendor arrangements, a consignment plan, a corporate prime vendor arrangement and a corporate prime vendor group purchasing arrangement. The vendor hopes that these many options will bring most of the business from the hospitals. But it seems that the number of national companies is decreasing, and through closings and mergers the number of regional and local companies is also growing smaller. If all medical-surgical companies but one or two major suppliers go out of business, this certainly would not be in the best interest of the hospitals.

Moreover, it is imperative that vendors and the health care industry and manufac-

Vendors and the health care industry and manufacturers must become involved in providing leadership to help hospitals reach the goal of cost containment and cost reduction while at the same time staying viable themselves.

turers become involved in providing leadership to help hospitals reach the goal of cost containment and cost reduction while at the same time staying viable themselves. This is the key in today's market. Would it ever be in the interest of the vendor to have a group of hospitals coalesce in order to get better prices? It probably would not be beneficial to the vendor unless the vendor's costs could be reduced in these group purchasing efforts.

The way group purchasing is structured today, hospitals want to be able to do away with back orders and at the same time get low prices. They do not want to build inventory, but they want to be able to get supplies on a few hours' notice. This has a detrimental effect on vendors by requiring them to keep large inventories and have more space available for these inventories.

In most cases, the only way the supplier or vendor can meet the goals of the group purchasing effort is to lower their own profits or shift the cost and expense to other hospitals not in the group. Group purchasing must seek the former solution.

There are several ways hospitals can help the vendor provide good prices, good service and lower costs. One way would be for the hospitals that participate in the group to warehouse the supplies at one central distribution point for the vendor. This would mean lower costs to the vendor, but it would most likely mean higher costs for the hospitals because they would have to duplicate their warehousing and distribution efforts. This would not be profitable for the hospital in the long run, and those groups that try to do it are being counterproductive.

Another way would be to have the vendor ship to each hospital at less frequent intervals, for example, once a month. This would cut down on transportation and distribution costs and would be helpful to the vendor. However, today's modern hospital purchasing agent sees a definite need to cut inventories and keep inventories at approximately a 14-day interval and turn them at least 26 times a year.

The vendor can cut costs by hiring fewer sales representatives, because the hospitals in a group purchasing association do not need to see a sales representative very often. Also, marketing and advertising are not as important and can be reduced under good purchasing efforts. Leadership from the vendors and suppliers is going to be more important in the future. The leadership must be assertive and help hospitals contain costs.

A GUIDE FOR NEGOTIATORS

Purchasing is a simple act that can be performed by automated means if necessary, but negotiation is an art. Really, group purchasing is a misnomer. One does not join a group purchasing endeavor simply to continue the same kind of purchasing that can be done by individual hospitals. The hospital joins a group to take advantage of group dynamics in the art of negotiation. Therefore, group purchasing directors and their staff should be the most experienced and effective negotiators for the entire group of hospitals.

In an effective group purchasing endeavor, the thrust must be toward skilled negotiation with the vendors. The vendors will not bow to a group just because it is a group. The vendors will soon know how much support is behind the group, and if it is a weak group with weak leadership, chances are the individual hospitals could do much better on their own.

A group contract cannot be negotiated in a day or two. To be most effective, group purchasing should aim for two- to three-year contracts. For example, if the hospital group is in a three-year contract, the director of group purchasing should begin negotiating the terms of the new contract at the beginning of the third year.

The needs of the hospitals

The director should make the terms of the contract as explicit as possible, and should put in writing all the terms of the proposed new contract except the prices; the various vendors who are asked to quote on the contract can fill in the prices. After the contract has been negotiated, purchasing would be the mere act of drawing on the terms of the group negotiations.

The purchasing group should have a clear idea of the prices they mean to pay for the various supplies proposed under the contract. To do that, the group should be responsible for comparing prices on a local, regional and national level. They should then review their past performance and commitment to group purchasing, which will give them some indication of how well they will make out in the negotiations. Such a review will also give the vendor an idea of what is in store and what is at stake.

There are other factors that will help hospitals in their materiel management endeavors. One factor is price protection. The group purchasing association should request and receive price protection on every line item that they purchase. Such protection may vary by line item, but should cover at least three months and as much as two years on some line items.

A maximum escalation clause should be part of the contract. On a three-year contract there should be almost no price changes in the first year, depending on the supply category for which one is negotiating. Then the group should put a maximum ceiling on price increases for the second year of 6 to 9 percent and the same maximum ceiling for the third year. Many purchasing groups do not consider price protection, and this has cost their groups many thousands of dollars.

In fact, with some supplies it is fairly easy to get price protection not for just a year but for a year and a half for the first phase. This kind of contract would be characteristic for I.V. solutions. However, if the group is negotiating for general medical-surgical supplies, price protection should be given for certain periods of time, for instance guaranteeing that there will be no price increases for 90 days and that there must be a written notice of at least 30 days before any price increases would be effective. Of course, the individual hospitals must agree to these prices.

> *The association between hospital and vendor is complex enough without having a separate transportation agency interjected into it, so the group should consider companies that have their own fleets of trucks and vans for delivery.*

Hospitals should not have to pay freight or delivery charges on any of the supplies. The group should give consideration to companies having their own fleet of trucks and vans for delivery. The association between hospital and vendor is complex enough without having a separate transportation agency interjected into it. So the group should ask for, if not insist on, a stable, consistent and predictable distribution system for their supplies, and in many cases this will involve vendor-owned transportation.

For some supply categories, there can be further negotiation for delivery and distribution of the goods to the hospitals. A good example of this is laundry service. If the hospital negotiating with an outside laundry has a cart distribution system for linen, the group purchasing director and the hospitals should try to have the purchasing price include the replenishment of the carts and distribution to the nursing units. If this kind of negotiation takes place, individual hospitals will be able to cut costs and get more services for fewer dollars.

The group should negotiate the scheduling of days and times for delivery of the supplies purchased under the contract. If each hospital provides times and days for the receipt of their goods and services, the vendor should be able to respond to these and work out a mutually satisfactory delivery schedule.

In this electronic and computerized age, the group would be remiss if it did not specify the kind of data input transmission that is necessary for all the hospitals to participate in the contract. The hospitals, if possible, should request a standard transmission system, which can range from data entry systems to manual systems. However, the group should specify the kind of information that the vendor would be responsible for providing to each individual hospital.

Vendors will guarantee their service levels and back them up with a penalty clause if hospitals require it. Hospitals should always request such a clause to take effect whenever the vendor does not perform to the service levels specified in the contract. Each hospital should be responsible for specifying order quantities and safety stock quantities for line items to be ordered under the contract. When the vendor has indicated that a sufficient amount of stock is in the warehouse to cover the hospital's normal ordering quantity plus the safety stock (usually one half of the normal ordering quantity), the hospital should insist on a penalty clause for nonperformance.

Payment terms are hardly ever part of group negotiations. The group should come to some understanding as to what the payment terms will be in the individual hospitals and use these terms in their negotiations. If the hospitals elect to pay the vendor twice per month, there should be considerations given by the vendor in return. In this time of high costs of money, the vendor certainly would be amenable to the negotiation of payment terms.

The vendor should be responsible for generating at least quarterly, if not monthly, reports on all the purchases by each hospital.

The needs of the vendor

Hospitals should provide the vendor with a total listing of items they are going to order under the contract and should indicate when the items will be needed. This helps vendors to forecast their needs and labor requirements.

If the group purchasing association has negotiated a tough contract, the vendor has the right to request prompt payment. This should be clearly stated in the contract. If the hospitals do not pay within the specified time period, a nonpayment penalty should be added to the outstanding balance. The vendor has a right to receive a copy of all hospital policies and procedures that pertain to the purchase, receipt and delivery of goods, payment of invoices and visits by salespeople.

To get a commitment from the vendor, the hospitals should make a commitment to order a certain volume of goods. If that volume is not ordered because of a change in the pattern of usage, then the contract should be amended. If, however, the agreed upon volume is not ordered because other vendors are getting the business, then the hospital should be prepared to pay a penalty to the vendor for violating the volume commitment.

Vendors usually speak in terms of volume, and hospitals speak in terms of the number of beds. The group pricing should be based on volume per bed per number of hospitals in the group. For example, a particular line item in the group purchasing price list may cost $4.50 when purchased in quantities of $1,200 per bed per year in a 2,000-bed group. This price would vary according to the volume per bed and the number of beds in the total purchasing group. Hospitals should put pressure on the vendor to offer group purchasing marketing and prices in terms the hospitals can understand.

COOPERATION AND COMMUNICATION

A common goal is a terrific motivator. Without one, there can be a lack of initiative and a failure to see the total picture. In group purchasing the goal should be the achievement of the best possible prices.

There must be good communication and cooperation among the hospitals, agents and vendors in order to achieve this goal. Too often agents fail to talk to each other and to the group purchasing director, and vendors complicate matters by carrying rumors back and forth. Group purchasing in many ways is an experiment in mutual trust.

Organizational structure and communication within the group should be kept simple. Hundred of thousands of dollars should not be spent to save $100,000. Group purchasing staffs should operate efficiently at low cost, and they should be reminded often that their main purpose is to save money for the patients of the hospitals they serve.

INCREASING THE EFFICIENCY OF GROUP PURCHASING

Product standardization is an excellent cost-containment technique. Hospitals with tough standardization programs operate very efficiently and should not be decentralized and fragmented by the group purchasing process. However, standardization and group purchasing are not mutually exclusive concepts. Group purchasing programs can be built around hospital standardization programs. With cooperation and consideration, this can be done easily.

Many hospitals are joining several groups and choosing the best prices among them. This is commonly referred to as "cherry picking." Groups must promote their prices and purchasing profiles in order to compete with other groups for excellence in purchasing. In fact, competition among groups may be the salvation of the entire group purchasing effort of the future.

The agent and director have several tools at their disposal to make group purchasing more effective. It is important to keep a statistical profile of exactly where the group has been, where it is now and where it intends to go. This would include statistics on line item volumes, usage by each hospital by line item, total dollar purchases by each hospital from each vendor, categorization of all line items in a priority listing from the most purchased to the least purchased, and annual price changes of line items.

Groups should share contractual arrangements on services. They should also encourage other groups by making avail-

able any information that will help the growth and maturation of another group. For example, they should make available price information. And it is important that groups use legitimate price comparisons. The *Aspen Hospital Purchasing Price Index* is an excellent tool for agents as well as groups. Hospitals and groups should participate in such a price index and share the information with each other on a quarterly basis. In this way, directors can profile and highlight any items that are out of line, and give praise where praise is due.

Directors and agents must get together on their position and not give away their strategy before the deal has been sealed or the contract has been let. There should be a penalty for agents who give out valuable information to vendors during the negotiation process. Communications must be strengthened among the hospitals and their parent organization. The more open the communications, the closer the bond among the hospitals. This will result in good prices and effective services for all hospitals.

Directors, with their agents, should develop a group master plan for the next three to five years. Such a plan should include a review of past experiences and a forecast of volumes, savings and extra services to be added in the future.

The successful group of the future will enter into the competitive market and maintain a marketing strategy to demonstrate and sell their capabilities and services. While the group is formulating a master plan, it should develop a catalog of the services that the group offers or intends to offer in the future. It should categorize all the contracts that are now available and describe any additional services it provides.

It is clear that group purchasing has worked, is working and will work in the future; however, the concept could be a lot more productive if purchasing group directors, hospital purchasing agents and vendors would make a real commitment to ensure meaningful participation beyond the token gestures that are now being called group purchasing.

REFERENCE

1. Housley, C.E., ed. *Aspen Hospital Purchasing Price Index* (Rockville, Md.: Aspen Systems Corp. 1981).

Group purchasing: past, present and future

Craig W. Moore
Vice President
Marketing and Business Development
American V. Mueller Division
American Hospital Supply Corporation
Chicago, Illinois

DOES GROUP PURCHASING represent the wave of the future or is it a
dinosaur heading for extinction? The
answer to that question depends primarily
on the negotiation process that will take
place between hospitals, vendors and
groups over the coming ten years. A look
at how group purchasing developed and
how it has handled challenges so far may
be helpful.

Group purchasing was first developed
for hospitals in the early 1900s. The first
group was the Hospital Bureau, Inc., in
Pleasantville, New York, founded in 1910.
Second was the Cleveland Hospital Association, formed in 1918. A third group, the
Joint Purchasing Corporation of New
York City, came into being about 1928. By
1962, 10 groups had been organized, and
between 1962 and 1974 an additional 40
groups were formed—bringing the total to
50 groups in 64 years. Between 1974 and
1977, the total number of groups in the
United States and Canada tripled.[1] Today

241

new groups continue to form and the old ones steadily expand.

Groups have been formed around government organizations such as federal, state, city and local procurement agencies; religious organizations; and other common considerations including geography. Additionally, there are the investor-owned hospital purchasing programs and the profit-making organizations which have hospital subscribers using their purchasing advantages.

The very marked increase in the number of groups from 1974 to 1977 can be attributed to federal and third party payer pressures to contain health care costs. Those costs represented approximately 8.8 percent of the GNP in 1978 and were projected to reach over 10 percent of the GNP by the early 1980s.[2] The Carter Administration's proposed 9 percent cap on hospital expenditures in 1977 gave further impetus to the expansion of group purchasing.

GROUP PURCHASING ACCOMPLISHMENTS TO DATE

Without question, these purchasing groups have given their hospitals a negotiating advantage. Many groups claimed savings well into the millions of dollars based on their contracts. Who benefited the most from these contracts? The answer must be qualified by type of benefit and by hospital size.

American Hospital Supply Corporation studies indicate 90 percent of the hospitals in the United States are members of at least one purchasing group. The greatest growth in purchasing group participation was among hospitals with less than 100 beds, especially those with 50 to 90 beds whose participation rose by 300 percent from 1970 to 1975. Large hospital (500-plus beds) participation grew less than 10 percent in the same period of time.[3]

Smaller hospitals would appear to have received the advantages of group purchasing through reduced prices. A secondary advantage could be found in a lightening of purchasing staff workload. Small hospitals purchase essentially the same products and services—although in less volume—as large hospitals. Their purchasing function is much the same, but must be performed with a substantially smaller staff. Group purchasing in small hospitals frees this limited work force considerably. Purchasing personnel are no longer overburdened with tasks such as vendor search and negotiation, and can turn their attention to other purchasing needs.

The larger hospitals benefited from group purchasing in two ways. The fact that they were members of groups certainly provided proof to anyone questioning their cost-containment efforts. Secondly, the large hospitals could point to their unit costs which were negotiated independently on the basis of their sheer dollar volume and/or prestige in the medical community and compare them to the published group costs.

GROUP PURCHASING PROBLEMS

While there have been gains made through group purchasing, there have also been problems. Groups are evaluated, in terms of power, by the number of beds they represent. Many groups therefore recruit large hospitals to add to their bed count. Because large hospitals have a reputation of reshopping the contract after it is signed, vendors often bid less aggressively, i.e., competitively, for the group contract.

To support the recruitment process, many groups have also expanded their contract programs. Initially, group contracts were for products that represented large dollars in the following categories: high volume and easily defined supplies, such as solutions or sutures; generic products such as drugs; products that hospitals accepted easily, such as fuel oil; and services such as laundry. Obviously, this was an expression of the famous 80/20 rule, where 80 percent of dollars are expended for 20 percent of products.

In the past several years, though, contracts have come to cover a far wider range of products. Some of the contracts are extremely broad, including thousands of items not readily standardized; surgical instruments or operating room supplies are good examples. These contracts are far more difficult to market. It is difficult to ensure that hospitals accept and comply with the contract agreements. While these contracts do provide savings, hospitals have problems in taking advantage of them because of the difficulties inherent in acquiring user approval. The groups become frustrated in marketing such contracts and, finally, vendors are disappointed at not receiving the desired results from the contracts. It is the consensus within the health care industry that these broad base contracts will be scaled down substantially in the 1980s.

Vendors are quickly recognizing that dual group memberships are weakening the ability of hospitals to make good on their volume commitments. Dual members will shop for contracts and eventually undercut the effectiveness of both groups. Secondly, the inability of some groups to productively market all of their contracts is creating supplier doubts about the effectiveness of groups. Consequently, suppliers today are less receptive to group contracts and are far more wary of the commitments groups make than they were ten years ago.

If suppliers retreat and the number of good supplier contracts drops, group

---

Dual group memberships are weakening the ability of hospitals to make good on their volume commitments. Dual members will shop for contracts and eventually undercut the effectiveness of both groups.

---

members will once again negotiate contracts independently. If this scenario develops, groups will find themselves in a negative spiral to extinction.

Groups today are also threatened by the improvements being made in individual hospital materiel management. Professional materiel managers, aided by computer systems, can run very effective programs for their hospitals. The efficiency of such programs and the strong administrative support it generates allow materiel managers to strengthen their commitments to suppliers; this places them in a preferred position against a group with limited ability to commit for its members.

In such circumstances, professional materiel managers will undoubtedly provide better cost-containment programs for their hospitals. Their buying commitment enables them to negotiate very good pricing but pricing still does not vary greatly between a group and a committed hospital contract. Where they really gain the advantage is through being in a better position to get the most out of the vendors' systems, services and inservices. These "secondary" advantages, which are built into every vendor's offer, are not marketed nearly as well by groups to the using departments as they are by materiel managers. The more comprehensive use by materiel managers of the warranties, inservices, etc., accompanying vendor offers results in the realization of a greater total savings.

LOOKING AHEAD: WHAT GROUPS NEED TO DO

In response to these problems, many groups are looking to group mergers to provide solutions as well as greater strength. Group mergers are not likely to be the way of the future, however. To serve a market effectively, it is necessary to be as close to it as possible. The decision making, the support and the commitments must be as close to the end user as possible. Furthermore, mergers cannot compensate for the inability of some groups to give their members a solid understanding of the volume they are bidding; generate

total membership commitment for their contracts; market their existing contracts effectively; or stop their bigger members from negotiating special agreements beyond that of the group contract. On the other hand, a group could enhance its negotiating position through the elimination of members who give only marginal support.

In a recent *Business Week* article, Chalmers predicts, "By the year 1990, the Americans will spend more on health care than the entire 1980 federal budget."[4] Genetic management could be a reality by then. The use of target drugs and other methods in treating diseases like cancer could substantially change surgery as we know it today. Preventive maintenance, health maintenance organizations and more attention to diets and physical fitness—all already under way—will dramatically change health care requirements. Demographic shifts will have an effect on where health care is delivered. That will include population shifts to the Sun Belt as well as shifts from hospitals to clinics and surgicenters. An increasing proportion of older persons will change the balance in type of care needed. And an older population, in an era of increased costs and new technology, will raise social and moral questions about strategies such as medical triage, which will be a far larger issue than abortion is today.

Depending on the success of for-profit health care institutions today, the health care industry will move toward domination by either for-profit institutions or by totally regulated nonprofit ones. Hospital consolidation and specialization will occur more frequently than they have to date.

How is the health care industry to deal successfully with the challenges facing it, and how does group purchasing fit into this picture? A number of recent publications—including *Business Week's* special issue on the reindustrialization of the United States[5] and Drucker's *Managing in Turbulent Times*[6]—have been devoted to the future and the kind of thinking that will be required from managers and organizations that intend to succeed in it. They all speak of the need for a new kind of strategic planning to ensure each success. The essence of the strategic planning will have to be around better negotiation of roles between hospital groups and vendors within the health care industry. These two groups will have to define more precisely the direction of the industry and negotiate the best utilization of their strengths in preparation for tomorrow's challenges.

The group purchasing industry can be expected to continue growing in the 1980s but group methods of operation will become more sophisticated and their services will expand beyond those of contract purveyors for quantity discount buying. Improved operational management between purchasing groups and members will result in higher dollar-per-bed commitments; therefore, there will be some additional improvements in pricing.

Committed volume contracts will increase as strengths develop. This will only happen in groups that understand the key requirements of their constituents and that know how to structure their contract agreements around those products and services they can effectively and efficiently market to their hospitals. In addition, there must be agreement, in advance, on the support they can expect from each member.

Price negotiation has already been much stressed; consequently, less remains to be gained in this area. The real potential gains for the 1980s are in the services, delivery systems and product quality that are to be had from vendors. To see that their hospitals get the best value, marketing staffs of groups must better understand what hospital needs are and what a vendor's total offer is in each istance.

The various relationships involved in group purchasing must take on a more

> **The real potential group purchasing gains for the 1980s are in the services, delivery systems and product quality that are to be had from vendors.**

cooperative and less adversary aspect. More time will be spent negotiating respective roles—of individual hospitals, groups and vendors—in health care. These discussions will include such areas as consulting services, delivery and storage, new products and systems developments. Negotiations will have to reach a much deeper understanding of each participant's concerns and interests in order to meet the requirements of tomorrow.

Most importantly, there must be projections for the future and discussion-negotiation of how respective roles will evolve to meet that future successfully. It is only in this way that group purchasing will play its part in helping the health care system meet the coming changes and challenges.

REFERENCES

1. American Hospital Supply Corporation. *Group Purchasing Now and in the 1980s* (Linden, N.J.: AHSC 1979).
2. Ibid.
3. Ibid.
4. Chalmers, T.C. and Stern, A.R. "Ideas and Trends." *Business Week* (February 23, 1981) p. 19.
5. Chalmers, T.C. "The Re-Industrialization of America—The Problem-A Solution-Will it Work?" *Business Week* special ed. (June 30, 1980).
6. Drucker, P.F. *Management in Turbulent Times* (New York: Harper & Row 1980).

Group purchasing: a vendor's perspective

Oren M. Williams, Jr.
Executive Vice-President
Nashville Surgical, Inc.
Nashville, Tennessee

THE CONCEPT of group purchasing is not new in the health care industry. It may come as a surprise to some of you to realize that group purchasing was a much discussed subject during the 1920s.

Today the United States has over 170 separate health care group purchasing organizations. A listing of them will reveal that they are everywhere and encompass all manner of activities.

The fact is simply that markets never change—they just shift. Here is a list of types of purchasing groups existing today in the United States:

- federation: a cluster of small groups;
- geographic: a council type (e.g., New England Purchasing Council);
- religious groups: (e.g., Daughters of Charity and Seventh-Day Adventists);
- government: Veterans Administration and federal hospitals under General Services Administration buying contracts;
- proprietary: (e.g., Hospital Corporation of America, Hospital Affiliates, International, Humana and Huma-

nex—proprietary groups which are 38 in number and growing);

- fraternal groups: (e.g., Shriner's Hospital and Screen Guild Hospitals);
- consortium groups: (e.g., Jewish Hospital Consortium and Sun Alliance, large hospitals [500 beds and over]);
- shared services (e.g., Western Kentucky Hospital Services which covers Mid and Western Kentucky and offers a laundry-drug-materiel management program and group purchasing contracts to members).

The foregoing shows the broad range of diversified accounts that are presently in the marketplace, all trying in their own right to cut hospital and patient end costs.

The importance of groups in today's health care is also reflected in projections that by the end of the decade in 1990: 85 percent of all general beds will be under some sort of group domain; 70 percent of all nursing home beds will be under some sort of group domain; and proprietary for-profit hospitals will continue to grow (they now control 10 percent of 7,000 hospitals and are on the move, acquiring more hospitals daily).[1,2]

How can vendors in the health care market survive in this environment? In trying to answer this question, it is useful to look at where hospitals buy and at how they buy. It is also important to remember that the cost of a product has three elements: cost of manufacture, cost of distribution and materiel management cost.

WHERE HOSPITALS BUY

Hospitals buy either from manufacturers (direct sellers) or from distributors. The two sources have distinctly different characteristics and methods.

Buying from manufacturers

Manufacturers or direct sellers *must* provide delivery, normally with maximum dollar order quantities; maintain research and development; maintain distribution points throughout the United States; and provide technical advice and knowledge on the use of their products. They must also invoice merchandise to hospital or group—this is normally a minimum invoice amount with penalties built in if invoice falls below certain parameters—and provide credit. Direct sellers normally demand and get payment within 45 days. If there is no payment, there is no shipment—and no shipment equals a credit hold. Terms are usually net 30 days or 1 percent 10th Prox.

Manufacturers must make a profit—the dirty word that has plagued so many throughout the health care field. Direct sellers or manufacturers normally reap about 25 to 65 percent gross profit margin. Direct sellers or manufacturers provide no emergency delivery except for an exorbitant special fee. The buyer who has pleaded for immediate action on holidays and weekends knows there is no such thing.

Buying through distributors

Distributors are accused by many of creating a large share of rising health costs in the United States. What in fact is their function?

Distributors and middlemen are essential in a country the size of the United

States and having such widely distributed facilities—7,099 hospitals with 1,407,097 beds in 50 states in 3,700 towns and cities.[3] These facilities, for the most part, rely on the middleman or distributor to provide them fluids, food, linens and other supplies for their day-to-day operations.

Medical distributors help to keep goods alive and costs down for these hospitals by providing warehousing—storing, stocking, rotating, accounting for traceability and handling recalls. They provide freight-out or delivery according to when the hospital

---

Medical distributors help to keep goods alive and costs down for hospitals by providing warehousing, freight-out or delivery, money, knowledgeable salespersons and manufacturer access.

---

wants it, where and in what quantity—for the most part with no minimum order, no add-on freight charge, no fuel surcharge and no administrative charges. And distributors provide *money*. They carry the load—no credit holds, no CODs. But with money costing 17 to 19.5 percent to borrow, money and cash flow mean survival, survival with a capital "S," for just in the last 3 years 14 distributors have thrown in the towel. Some might say they simply could not manage properly. This may be partly true but also greatly to blame were inadequate cash flow and nonpayment of bills.

Distributors provide salespersons. These individuals travel throughout the country, providing a valuable and sometimes much

maligned service. They introduce new products, transfer product knowledge and problem-solving expertise, and create liaison between hospitals and manufacturers. Such salespeople are not going to become extinct, but will be used more fully in the future as providers and as the communications arm of distributors. They should not be treated like the "rack breadmen" in a grocery store.

Finally, distributors offer a clearinghouse or umbrella for groups by providing access to many manufacturers. For example, an Alabama distributor acts as intermediary for 32 separate manufacturers with 900 items on contract to one buying group. Suppose each buying group had to handle the administrative load that is being created because of more contracts, more members, more items and fewer middlemen or distributors who are operating on less profit dollar.

The forbidden word—profit—has just been mentioned again. Distributors too must make a profit. They are "for profit." They pay taxes and must make money. The average surgical distributor who is also a health care provider works on an operating cost of 12 to 13 percent gross sales with a net bottom line profit of approximately 2 percent of gross sales after federal taxes. This profit margin is a great deal less than that of national distributor-manufacturer chains, whose overall gross margins are 2 to 5 times better. This difference has less to do with operating efficiencies than with the chains' marketing programs and their ability to manufacture restrictive, noncompetitive lines. The independent middleman is still the most economical means of health care product *delivery*.

HOW HOSPITALS BUY

Catch-as-catch-can

The first approach to buying may be described as "catch-as-catch-can." This can take the form of (a) *managerial anarchy*, everyone doing his or her own thing; (b) *management by crisis*, the department has plans, but no one sticks to them—they simply put out fires; (c) *by gosh-by golly approach*, "by gosh, I *guess* it's time to order some and by golly I better order a lot"; (d) *blanket order*, by educated guess; and (e) *true decision analysis*, a method giving the whole range of formulas for ordering which is a true logical sequence (economic order quantity is an example).

Each of these affects the cost of goods procured. The only rational approach is true decision analysis. A distributor cannot function satisfactorily unless the buying group itself reaches certain management goals and guidelines in relation to how to order goods. When hospital management does its buying on a catch-as-catch-can basis, it is difficult for the middleman to produce.

Individual purchasing contracts

Another method of purchasing is through an individual hospital contract. This approach is still common and offers certain tried pros and cons. On the positive side, individual hospital contracts are easy to administer, their prices are generally competitive with those of hospitals in the same area and there is little change in product usage (in other words, each product line that is well accepted is bid yearly).

On the other hand, due to small volume, prices to individual hospitals must usually be higher than to groups. Also, for the most part, the manufacturers who establish national price trends will not do much for a small 60-bed hospital on an individual contract. And with an individual contract, price protection is limited, materiel management usage reports are limited and there are no penalty clauses.

Prime vendor contracts

A third buying approach is the prime vendor contract. Such agreements have been the subject of many articles exalting their pros and their cons. In the Aspen Corporation's 1980 report on the functions of the prime vendor contract, Patters of the General Accounting Office took the position "that Prime Vendor contracts do not save you money, and I would not recommend going to the Prime Vendor concept from an accounting standpoint."[4]

On the other side of the fence, two well-known and published advocates of hospital materiel management and prime vendor contracts are Ammer and Housley. Ammer has said, "Everyone wins . . . with a systems contract that is awarded competitively."[5] And, according to Housley, "In order to promise enough volume to make negotiations worthwhile to the supplier, the prime vendor is recommended; and I think this concept is best for the Hospital in the long and short range."[6]

Group purchasing

Last but not least is group contract or group purchasing. The jury is still out on this method of buying. However, increasing government control and the tightening up of Medicare reimbursement should bring its advantages and disadvantages into sharper focus.

According to the American Surgical Trade Association there is a widespread assumption that group purchasing operations provide savings to hospitals that participate in them. However, considerable evidence is beginning to emerge that many of the claims for group purchasing savings are highly inflated. In many cases, immediate savings may be outweighed by the administrative costs of the program or by other expenses, such as the cost of

---

In many cases, the immediate savings due to group purchasing are outweighed by the administrative costs of the program or by other expenses, such as the cost of increased inventory.

---

increased inventory, that must be incurred by hospitals purchasing medical supplies through a shared services organization.[7]

The Health Resources Administration in 1976 financed a $1.6 million project of the Productivity Center of the Texas Hospital Association to study ways to reduce costs of hospital operations. This study led to two finished documents: a "Literature Review of Group Purchasing" and a book titled *Cheaper by the Dozen? A Guide to Group Purchasing.*

"Increased buying power often reduces the price per item obtained by the group members. However, the reduction in price per unit may be absorbed and even outweighed by additional materials management costs."[8] A General Accounting

Office (GAO) study found that in 5 of 6 cities surveyed membership in group purchasing associations did not necessarily result in hospitals getting the lowest prices available in the area. For example, in Cincinnati and Columbus, when prices the groups paid for the items surveyed were compared to the prices paid by other hospitals in the area, only about 40 percent of the items obtained by groups were acquired at the lowest prices. And about 5 percent of the items contracted by the groups were at the highest price.

In Seattle, group purchasing arrangements resulted in hospitals getting the lowest price for about 45 percent of the items. Furthermore, in the one city (Pittsburgh) where the GAO found that the group purchasing organization was providing the lowest price for the majority (63 percent) of the items surveyed, the price savings were not substantial, since "the area prices surveyed tended to cluster around the group price."[9]

The main function of group purchasing organizations to date had been simply one of negotiating a contract; after that, delivery to the hospital and billing are handled directly by the supplier. Where most group prices are lower, it is usually because the contracts negotiated have been devoid of services and deal for the most part with large-volume items.

For a hospital to pay as much for products that come to it without services as another hospital in the same community pays for products that come with services discriminates against the very supplier who is probably making the greatest contribution to cost control. The result would be a variation of the economists' axiom that "bad money drives out good"; if the effective charge for poor quality goods without services becomes the same as for higher quality goods with services, the quality of goods and services will decline.

Groups and group administrators should not try to rely on price and price alone as the one key point in negotiations.

If they do, groups will wind up with fewer vendors bidding, lower levels of service and generally poor quality goods.

The jury is indeed still out, but hospitals and vendors should work together—not against each other—to keep health care quality up and costs down.

REFERENCES

1. Sandomir, R. "Profitable Revolution." *Financial World* (February 15, 1981) p. 43–46.

2. Sherwood Irwen, "Report to the Mid-Western Hospital Council." Paper delivered to the Hospital Council, March 1981, under the auspices of the United Hospital Supply Corporation, Chicago, Illinois.

3. American Hospital Association. *Statistical Data Sheet* (Chicago: AHA 1981).

4. Patters cited in Bartlett, W.M., "The Future of Prime Vendor Concept." *Hospital Materiel Management Quarterly* 2:1 (1980) p. 35–42.

5. Ammer, D.S., *Purchasing and Materials Management for Health Care Institutes* (Lexington, Mass.: Lexington Books 1975) p. 31.

6. Housley, C.E., *Hospital Materiel Management* (Germantown, Md.: Aspen Systems Corp. 1978) p. 208

7. Robert Anderson, President, American Surgical Trade Association, Chicago (in a letter to Administrator, HCFA-HEW, October 16, 1978).

8. Texas Hospital Association. *Cheaper by the Dozen: A Hospital Guide to Group Purchasing* (Austin: THA 1980) p. 78.

9. Thomas Bloor, President, American Surgical Trade Association, Chicago (in a letter to Administrator, HCFA-HEW, May 1, 1980).

Minimizing the antitrust risks of group purchasing

Richard S. Lovering, M.B.A., J.D.
Bricker & Eckler
Columbus, Ohio

GROUP PURCHASING is a tool for cost containment that no hospital administration can afford to ignore. The American Hospital Association has noted 38 different services which may be shared on a multi-institutional level.[1] Besides purchasing, shared services include data processing, food services, garbage collection, laundry, blood banking, diagnostic radiology and emergency medical services. Suppliers benefit from shared services because unit costs are reduced as the result of economies of scale and because committed volume permits a reduction in the suppliers' risk. Hospitals benefit from reduced costs because of increased bargaining power, lower inventory costs as the result of standardization, consolidated purchasing administration and savings passed on by suppliers. With proper antitrust compliance planning, these benefits can be enjoyed by suppliers and hospitals with a minimized risk of antitrust exposure.

POTENTIAL ANTITRUST RISKS

All collective activities by a group of competitors raise the specter of an antitrust violation. By the creation of the group the members have satisfied the contract, combination or conspiracy requirement of section 1 of the Sherman Act. Group activities by competitors in the health care industry are especially dangerous.

As recently noted by the chairman of the Health Care Committee of the Antitrust Law Section of the American Bar Association, five times as many health antitrust actions have been brought since 1975 than during the previous 85 years of the Sherman Act.[2] Because the health care industry has a history of collective activities and because it is perceived by the public to be riddled with inflated costs, it makes a politically attractive target for scrutiny by the Justice Department and Federal Trade Commission. The prospect of treble damages provides a continuing incentive for private plaintiffs to test the legality of multi-institutional activities.

Traditional health care industry exemptions from the antitrust laws are under attack. Recently the state action exemption and McCarran-Ferguson Act exemptions were eroded in *California Retail Liquor Dealers Ass'n v. Midcal Aluminum,* 445 U.S. 97 (1980), and *Group Life & Health Insurance Co. v. Royal Drug Co.* 440 U.S. 205 (1979), respectively. The implied exemption for activities voluntarily supportive of the policies of the National Health Planning and Resources Develop-

Despite their fundamental compatibility of purpose, antitrust laws and group purchasing may come into conflict because the antitrust laws view skeptically all group activities by actual or potential competitors.

ment Act of 1974 was eliminated by the Supreme Court ruling in *National Gerimedical Hospital v. Blue Cross of Kansas City,* 452 U.S. 378 (1981). The area is currently very volatile. In short, all group activities in the health care industry should be undertaken with extreme care and advance planning to minimize the antitrust risks.

Ostensibly, the antitrust laws and group purchasing have the same purpose. Most antitrust economists would agree that the purpose of the antitrust laws is to ensure the existence of a competitive marketplace where the consumer benefits from prices reduced by the rigors of competition. The purpose of group purchasing is to reduce the cost of goods and services to health care facilities. Despite their fundamental compatibility of purpose, antitrust laws and group purchasing may come into conflict because the antitrust laws view skeptically all group activities by actual or potential competitors.

Purchasing groups should be aware of the danger of violating sections 1 and 2 of the Sherman Act and section 2(f) of the Robinson-Patman Act. (See Appendix.) These acts are complemented by the Federal Trade Commission Act, nearly a century of antitrust case law, and similar state antitrust statutes.

Section 1 of the Sherman Act: Price Fixing

The usual antitrust rules against restraints of trade apply to hospital shared services. Therefore group purchasing efforts cannot be used to restrict price competition, divide markets, boycott suppliers or boycott another health care provider.

In the classic price fixing decision, *United States v. Socony-Vacuum Oil Co.,* 315 U.S. 150 (1940), the Supreme Court stated, "a combination formed for the purpose and with the effect of raising, depressing, fixing, pegging, or stabilizing the price of a commodity in interstate or foreign commerce is illegal." In *Kiefer-Steward Co. v. Joseph E. Seagram & Sons,* 340 U.S. 211 (1951), the court decided that an agreement among competitors setting maximum prices is also a violation of section 1.

Group purchasing may contribute to a uniformity of hospital rates in an area because all hospitals in the group may have the same cost for supplies and because the supplier's price to the group may act as a floor on rates in a given market area. If a uniform rate structure between hospitals results, there could be an appearance that rates had been fixed. In addition, common membership in a purchasing group could promote communication between hospital administration in which prohibited discussions on hospital rates or territories take place.

To avoid the broad scope of *Socony-Vacuum,* members of a hospital purchasing group must be zealous not to permit the stabilization and uniformity of costs to the purchasing group to become the basis for formal or informal agreements with the purpose and effect of establishing uniform rates between competing hospitals. Each hospital must continue to set its rates solely on the basis of its own administration's independent business judgment. Absolutely no communications should be made with competitors concerning territories or rates. A third person who is not a competitor, such as an attorney, a secretary or friend, should be privy to all conversations with competitors.

Group boycotts

Another potential antitrust pitfall of group purchasing is the possible allegation of group boycott. The classical group boycott has been defined as a concerted effort to induce suppliers or customers to withhold their trade from a competitor of the concerted group in order to make it impossible for the competitor to compete.[3] The possibility of an illegal group boycott in the group purchasing context is twofold. First, a group boycott could exist at the hospital level because a specific health care provider had been excluded from the purchasing group. Second, a group boycott could exist at the supplier level because a competing supplier had been foreclosed from the market consisting of the members of the purchasing group.

Boycott at the hospital level

If nonmembership in the purchasing group places a competitor at a significant competitive disadvantage, then all membership criteria in the purchasing group must be objective and in no way designed to exclude a particular competitor. Malcolm MacArthur suggests that membership in a purchasing group must be available to all members of an industry.[4] As the competitive benefits of membership become more vital to success in the industry, the consistency of objective membership criteria with the purposes of the group becomes more important.

For instance, criteria based on geographic location of the purchasing group members are acceptable if those criteria are related to concerns over the area a purchasing group can effectively service. However, under no circumstances should the purchasing group assign exclusive territories to its members or refuse membership to an entity because it is a competitor of an existing member.

Membership criteria based on size may also be suspect. If smaller purchasers are excluded from a purchasing group, they can allege that the large purchasers in the group by denying small purchasers the benefits of group membership were conspiring to restrain trade by interfering with the smaller purchasers' ability to compete.

Boycott at the supplier level

Hospital purchasing groups risk being implicated as co-conspirators in actions by disgruntled suppliers who have been foreclosed from a large market of several hospitals because a competing supplier obtained a contract with the purchasing group. The risk of this problem increases when the purchasing group represents a large number of hospitals in an area and when hospitals are major purchasers of the goods or service.

The major case in this area is *White & White, Inc. v. American Hospital Supply Corp.*, 540 F. Supp. 951 (1982). In that case, a group of suppliers alleged, among other things, that the American Hospital Supply Corporation (AHS) conspired to restrain trade with Voluntary Hospitals of America, Inc. (VHA), a purchasing organization for 29 of the nation's largest nonprofit hospitals. The plaintiffs claimed that AHS and VHA conspired to exclude the competing suppliers. In that case, Judge Hillman reasoned that hospital group purchasing is not necessarily prohibited by the antitrust laws. Nevertheless, a verdict of $430,638.00 was awarded against the defendants and the unique and complex purchase agreement in that case was held to constitute a conspiracy to restrain trade and an attempt to monopolize the hospital supply distribution business.

Since the court's decision in *White & White,* a federal district court in Georgia has upheld a VHA group purchasing agreement in *Langston Corp. v. Standard Register Co., et al.,* 553 F. Supp. 632 (N.D. Ga. 1982). In that case, VHA recommended a business forms supplier but did not require VHA hospitals to buy any of their forms from the recommended supplier. The court in that case recognized that group purchasing is a conventional means of reducing costs and that no anticompetitive motive could be presumed. On the facts of that case, the court refused to find an antitrust violation. Similarly, the Antitrust Division of the Department of Justice has issued a business review letter in which it indicated that it does not intend to challenge the group purchasing program of the Ohio Hospital Purchasing Consortium of Columbus, Ohio (OHPC). The OHPC plan provides that no participating hospital is required to purchase through OHPC or is prevented from dealing with any supplier.

To minimize the risks that excluded suppliers will allege group boycott or exclusive dealing. *White & White* and the subsequent cases indicate that supply contracts should affirmatively state that the contract does not preclude the purchasing group or individual member hospitals from purchasing from other suppliers. In addition, bids from as many potential suppliers as is practically possible should be solicited by the purchasing group. The criteria for determining which suppliers will be asked to bid should be objective factors such as geographic location and product characteristics. Similarly, criteria used for accepting bids should be objective and readily documented, such as price and quality.

Price discrimination under the Robinson-Patman Act

Many experienced practitioners—like George Hart of the Legal Affairs Department of the Washington Hospital Center and Malcolm MacArthur, a former trial attorney for the Antitrust Division of the U.S. Department of Justice—believe that the major antitrust pitfall of group purchasing arises under the Robinson-Patman Act[5,6] (see Appendix). The Robinson-Patman Act requires that favorable prices received by the buying group should be available to all competitors unless the price to the hospital was made to meet a competing supplier's price or was cost-justified. Section 2(f) of the Robinson-Patman Act provides that it is illegal for buyers to induce or receive a discriminatory price which is not covered by a defense of meeting competition or cost justification. Purchases by nonprofit institutions for their own use are exempt from the Robinson-Patman Act.

According to a recent ruling by the Supreme Court in *Great Atlantic & Pacific Tea Co. v. FTC*, 440 U.S. 69 (1979), a buyer cannot be liable under section 2(f) for inducing a seller to offer a discriminatory price if the seller is not liable for price discrimination. For a purchasing group it is a defense to a section 2(f) claim that its supplier had a cost justification for discriminating in price in the buying group's favor. Such a cost justification could consist of the cost savings enjoyed by a supplier because of the high volume purchases by the purchasing group. Similarly, the purchasing group could assert as a defense to a section 2(f) claim that the discriminatory price was offered by the seller in a good faith attempt to meet the lower price of a competing supplier.

To minimize the risk of a Robinson-Patman Act violation, membership in the purchasing group should be available to all competitors who meet the bona fide objective membership criteria of the group. In addition, if the buying group attempts to induce a supplier to meet a competing supplier's price, the buying group should document the meeting competition defense by obtaining written documentation of the first supplier's price.

GUIDELINES FOR AVOIDING ANTITRUST SUITS

As a general rule, no communications should be made with competitors concerning rates, territories or any other factors affecting competition, and a third person who is not a competitor should be privy to all conversations with competitors.

Membership criteria should be objective and based on demonstrable commercial necessity.

Members should be free to purchase supplies independently and should not be obligated to commit themselves to the purchasing group for the exclusive purchase of their supplies. The agreement between the purchasing group and the member hospitals should affirmatively state that member hospitals retain the right to bargain freely with all suppliers in the marketplace.

The purchasing group should not be a party to a contract with a supplier which conditions the sale of goods on an explicit or implicit understanding by the purchasing group or its members that they will not purchase products from competing suppliers. In addition, supply contracts should be subject to periodic rebidding.

The purchasing group should solicit bids from as many suppliers as is feasible, and should use objective factors, such as price and product characteristics, in determining which bid to accept.

Price differentials given to the group, directly or in the form of a rebate, should be either based on cost savings to the supplier or based on a good faith effort by the supplier to meet the price of a competing supplier. If the price differential is based on an effort to meet a competing seller's price, the purchasing group should document the competing seller's bid by getting a copy of that bid in writing.

These precautions will lessen the likelihood of a purchasing group or its member hospitals being involved in an antitrust suit. If the purchasing group or its member hospitals do become involved in an antitrust suit, the contract clauses, operating procedures and record-keeping practices recommended here could aid in the defense of the case.

Purchasing groups in the health care industry are a potential source of considerable cost savings in the health care industry. With proper advance compliance planning and consultation with legal counsel, the antitrust risks of group purchasing can be minimized.

REFERENCES

1. AHA study quoted in the presentation of P. Proger on shared service organizations at the Fourth Annual Program on Antitrust in the Health Care Field, Washington, D.C., January 7, 1981. See also Proger, P.A. "Antitrust and Shared Services" in *Antitrust in the Health Care Field* (Towson, Md.: National Health Pub. 1979) p. 169.
2. Halper, H.R. "The Health Care Industry and the Antitrust Laws." 49 ABA Antitrust L.J. 17 (1981) p. 17.
3. Sullivan, L. *Handbook of the Law of Antitrust* (St. Paul, Minn.: West Publishing 1977) §83–84.
4. MacArthur, M. *Associations and the Antitrust Laws* (U.S. Chamber of Commerce, Washington, D.C. 1976) p. 63.
5. Hart, G. Legal Affairs Dept., Washington Hospital Center, Washington, D.C. Personal Communication, June 1981.
6. MacArthur. *Associations and the Antitrust Laws.* p. 63.

SHERMAN ACT, 15 U.S.C. §1

Section 1 of the Sherman Act provides in relevant part:

[E]very contract, combination ... or conspiracy, in restraint of trade or commerce among the several States, or with foreign nations, is hereby declared to be illegal. Every person who shall make any contract or engage in any combination or conspiracy hereby declared to be illegal shall be deemed guilty of a felony and, on conviction thereof, shall be punished by fine not exceeding one million dollars if a corporation, or, if any other person, one hundred thousand dollars, or by imprisonment not exceeding three years, or by both said punishments, in the discretion of the court.

SHERMAN ACT, 15 U.S.C. §2

Section 2 of the Sherman Act provides in relevant part:

[E]very person who shall monopolize, or attempt to monopolize, or combine or conspire with any other person or persons, to monopolize any part of the trade or commerce among the several States, or with foreign nations, shall be deemed guilty of a felony, and, on conviction thereof, shall be punished by fine not exceeding one million dollars if a corporation, or, if any other person, one hundred thousand dollars, or by imprisonment not exceeding three years, or by both said punishments, in the discretion of the court.

ROBINSON-PATMAN ACT, 15 U.S.C. §13

The Robinson-Patman Act provides in relevant part:

Sec. 2(a) [T]hat it shall be unlawful for any person engaged in commerce ... to discriminate in price between different purchasers of commodities of like grade and quality, ... where the effect of such discrimination may be substantially to lessen competition or tend to create a monopoly in any line of commerce, or to injure, destroy, or prevent competition with any person who either grants or knowingly receives the benefit of such discrimination, or with customers of either of them: Provided, that nothing herein contained shall prevent differentials which make only due allowance for differences in the cost of manufacture, sale, or delivery resulting from the differing methods or quantities in which such commodities are to such purchasers sold or delivered.

(b) Upon proof being made, at any hearing on a complaint, under this section, that there has been discrimination in price or services or facilities furnished, the burden of rebutting the prima facie case thus made by showing justification shall be upon the person charged with a violation of this section, and unless justification shall be affirmatively shown, the Commission is authorized to issue an order terminating the discrimination: Provided, however, that nothing herein contained shall prevent a seller rebutting the prima facie case thus made by showing that his lower price or the furnishing of services or facilities to any purchaser or purchasers was made in good faith to meet an equally low price of a competitor, or the services or facilities furnished by a competitor.

(f) That it shall be unlawful for any person engaged in commerce, in the course of such commerce, knowingly to induce or receive a discrimination in price which is prohibited by this section.

Selecting the right group purchasing program

Jack Anderson
Program Director
Council Shared Services, Inc.
Los Angeles, California

IN MANY AREAS of the United States, a hospital has the luxury of selecting from two or more group purchasing organizations. This opportunity allows purchasing or materiel managers to choose the group best equipped to meet the needs of the hospital and most complementary to the manager's own abilities.

Selecting a purchasing group is not unlike choosing a spouse. The parties should be compatible and share similar interests and goals. It is important to develop mutual trust and respect, and both parties must be willing to grow together in sickness and in health, good times and bad. Mutual commitment to each other's success and welfare will bring about a lasting relationship.

Selecting the best group purchasing program for you is important to your personal performance as well as the prices your hospital pays for its goods and services. You are delegating some of your negotiating duties to another buyer—in this case, a buyer who does not report directly to you. The selection of the right candidate for this key position requires a thorough evaluation of all the options available.

NONVOLUNTARY PURCHASING GROUPS

Group purchasing was first applied by hospitals sharing a commonality of ownership, both public and private. The Veterans Administration, hospitals sharing a religious affiliation, state institutions and proprietary health care organizations have all consolidated their purchases for the purpose of reducing their costs.

Most of these proprietary hospitals would not elect to join a voluntary group purchasing organization, even though some contracts written by a voluntary group are better than those negotiated by the owners of their hospital. Clearly, hospitals with a commonality of ownership feel that supporting their association of hospitals is more important than the higher prices they may be paying. This consideration and the anticipation of more and better contracts in the future keep many of these hospitals out of voluntary purchasing groups.

It must be noted that proprietary, religious and government hospitals invariably write group procurement agreements and frequently cite these contracts as a primary benefit for owned hospitals. This fact should be a strong message to the timid people who doubt the benefits to be derived from participation in purchasing groups.

CRITERIA FOR SELECTING A PURCHASING GROUP

Type of organization

A purchasing group may be sponsored by nonprofit associations, such as a state or county hospital association, or it may be an independent nonprofit or for-profit organization. For example, one large purchasing group in the west is a private company which operates for profit and is unaligned with any state, regional or proprietary organization, and does not perform contract services to state and regional associations.

The type of organization may not matter to you at all, or may be a factor only if other criteria are equal. Conversely, if your hospital administration is a strong supporter of a regional or state hospital association with a group purchasing program, your participation in an unaffiliated group may be precluded.

A regional purchasing group may be affiliated with other organizations to form a "super group." This larger group may be able to negotiate more favorable agreements than those available to the individual members. It would be wise to determine whether the groups you are considering belong to a super group to avail your hospital of the benefits and potential benefits of these ventures.

Contractual commitment

The operations of various purchasing groups can be distinguished by the type of contract they write, which can be broadly summarized as committed or noncommitted.

Committed contracts ensure for the vendor the purchased volume of the participating hospitals and are apt to receive the most favorable pricing since vendors compete in a win-or-lose contest. In order to participate in a committed volume purchasing program, purchasing or materiel managers must be able to sell their hospitals on the contract brand. Some groups hedge on the committed volume contract by establishing dual vendors for each item. This may make the task of complying with the contract easier for the purchasing agent since the product choices have doubled. The dual vendor suppliers still have some assurance that their sales will increase, and their prices should reflect this expectation. Dual vendor prices should not be expected to be as low as in the single vendor agreements, where a supplier is faced with an all-or-nothing situation.

Noncommitted purchasing contracts require no indication from a hospital of an intent to participate in the agreement. Vendors are simply offering a price in anticipation of increased business, often encouraged by the group purchasing director. The advantage of this style of contracting is that the hospital's purchasing manager does not have to accept specific contract brands. Instead, purchasing agents can ask the group to enter into an agreement with the manufacturer preferred by their hospital. In addition, noncommitted purchasing groups claim that hospitals are able to buy a greater percentage of their needs from group contracts and no hospital is excluded from using agreements because it prefers another brand.

The disadvantage of noncommitted groups is the prices they pay. Why should a supplier offer a discount on existing business when additional sales volume is not assured? A company may be enticed into cutting prices for a year or so, but the "carrot on the end of a stick" approach

---

The disadvantage of noncommitted groups is the prices they pay. Why should a supplier offer a discount on existing business when additional sales volume is not assured?

---

can work only for so long. Sooner or later, the vendor will want increased sales volume in return for discounted prices.

Participation in contracting

Some group purchasing organizations involve their members in deciding what to contract and where to solicit bids; the ultimate contract acceptance or rejection is voted on by the members. Other purchasing groups occasionally survey their members as to their desires but write agreements without the direct involvement of the hospital representatives. The best group for you may be the one that suits your objectives and personality. If you like to be involved in negotiations and feel you have something to offer the group, a participatory group is for you. On the other hand, if you would rather delegate this task or cannot regularly attend meetings because of the distance or your time schedule, you may be happier with a nonparticipating program.

When a group is writing committed

volume contracts, the participation of the members is essential. Not only are vendor approvals and volume commitments required from the members, but the involvement of the members in establishing a contract creates enthusiasm and support for the program. Purchasing and materiel managers encourage each other and share their experiences with product lines and vendors and become strong advocates for their particular purchasing group.

Range of activities and prices

An evaluation of purchasing groups does not end with a price comparison of the most common medical–surgical supplies. Many purchasing groups have programs for pharmacy, laboratory, dietary, housekeeping, maintenance and office supplies as well as fuel and medical gases. Some groups have established shared computer programs for inventory and purchasing and have negotiated biomedical repair contracts as well as service agreements for office equipment. You should not overlook the agreements available for the more common capital equipment items such as office furniture, intravenous pumps and patient monitors.

The range of group purchasing applications is limited only by one's imagination and time. Look for a group that is aggressively expanding its scope of activities.

Paying a lower price for goods and services is the principal reason for the existence of group purchasing organizations, so comparing the prices of the groups being considered is essential to the selection process. The price survey should include data on the length of contracts with price protection clauses, any delivery,

handling and minimum order charges, and any other information you would request from any other supplier. You should note how many contracts are available through the group from manufacturers currently being used, since great prices will not help if the brand is unacceptable to your hospital. Moreover, implementing the savings from your purchasing group participation will be faster and easier if you minimize the number of product line changes.

You should be aware that the representative prices you receive from a purchasing group will be tailored to show its performance in the most favorable light. The shopping list for your hospital will vary, so create your own list of high-volume items for price comparison.

Number of beds in participating hospitals

Suppliers trade lower prices for increased volume, so it stands to reason that the greater the volume, the lower the prices. When there is a high level of commitment to the group contract on the part of the member hospitals, a purchasing group can wield a great deal of influence with manufacturers, and the contract should reflect the commitment through lower prices. A moderate-sized group with poor participation will pay higher prices than a smaller group with strong group commitment.

One particularly large hospital supplier proposes to offer different group prices to each hospital on a dollars-per-bed basis. Their rationale is that the percent of overhead is related to sales volume. Higher volume allows the supplier to maintain the existing profit margin while reducing prices. Under this plan large purchasing groups have no advantage over smaller ones and prices bid by other vendors are difficult to compare because this large supplier charges each hospital in the group a different price (base price less a variable discount). If this sounds like a divide-and-conquer ploy to you, you're right! Competition between manufacturers is less keen and group members lose their cohesiveness. The group effectiveness and unity can be maintained if uniform volume incentives are contracted for all participating hospitals.

It is more cost effective to purchase some commodities locally. To obtain these items through group purchasing methods the group would have to establish several regional contracts for the same commodity or limit the selection to a local purchasing group.

Some purchasing groups contract with dealers who do not serve customers outside a limited area. Clearly, the purchasing group must make an effort to arrange for service to member hospitals in outlying areas.

With the increased activity by super groups, the health care marketplace will become more national than regional in character. Group purchasing clients can benefit from the formation of large groups if continuity of service from suppliers can be assured.

Fee structure

The manner in which group purchasing organizations derive revenue to sustain their operations will vary among groups. Some popular fee structures are:

1. fixed fee for total program;
2. fixed fee per selected programs;
3. fixed fee per bed;
4. fixed fee per patient day;
5. percentage of hospital purchases (paid by the hospital); and
6. percentage of sales to group (paid by the vendor).

The fee is usually insignificant compared to the savings that are obtained, but most prudent purchasing managers are concerned about getting full value for every dollar spent. No one wants group purchasing fees to be mismanaged or a for-profit purchasing group to receive an excessive profit. We can compare fees among groups and measure these differences against the savings realized; however, after several years of involvement with a group, it is difficult to calculate the costs you would be paying to vendors if you were not a group participant.

One way to evaluate fees is to calculate the percentage of total contract dollars they represent. A group with $2 million in contracts and a total fee revenue of $50,000 is operating at 2.5 percent of contract dollars. In private for-profit groups where the financial statistics are not available, you can divide your hospital's fees by the anticipated purchases to derive this percentage. A rule of thumb for a reasonable group purchasing fee is 1 percent of the contract purchases. Groups just beginning or those with ancillary services, such as time-shared computers, would be somewhat higher.

Information sharing

Do the purchasing groups you are evaluating share price and contract information with other groups? If they do, they are learning valuable information about successes and failures in other parts of the country. You may ask the purchasing group representatives if their organization belongs to the Group Purchasing Group, an association made up of local and regional purchasing groups throughout the country. A purchasing group in regular contact with other similar organizations is likely to be working actively to improve its services to members.

Hospital personality

The climate within your particular hospital may be a factor in selecting a group purchasing organization. Is "hospital personality" another name for politics? Yes and no. Certainly you should be supportive of a purchasing group sponsored by your state hospital association when your administrator is the president of the organization. But it is also prudent to objectively evaluate your ability to effect change within your institution. If your hospital staff is receptive to change and to cost-containment efforts, you are likely to achieve good results in a committed volume purchasing group. Conversely, if change is strongly resisted, it may be wise to join a noncommitted organization.

The size of your hospital and any specialized services that are offered also affect its personality. The purchasing group you select should have other members of approximately the same size. Vendors bidding for a contract must factor the cost of servicing each account into their prices, and a large hospital may not improve its pricing by joining a purchasing group made up of very small units.

Specialized hospitals, such as pediatric facilities or burn centers, should look for purchasing groups that represent other hospitals with a similar specialty, since these purchasing groups are more likely to develop contracts for the specialized products used by these institutions.

MAKING YOUR SELECTION

You will undoubtedly be able to think of additional factors for selecting the right purchasing program. The task of weighing the relative importance of these various factors is much more difficult, and, returning to the analogy of marriage again, it is most important that you consider the elements that are necessary to develop a lasting relationship—trust, respect and commitment to each other's success and happiness.

A hospital can belong to several purchasing groups—one for pharmaceuticals, medical–surgical and laboratory supplies, another for a food service program, a third for furniture and office equipment and still another for medical capital equipment.

It would be inadvisable to commit to two or more purchasing groups for the same supply items. The success of group purchasing is based on member support and commitment to the program. Suppliers offer lower prices to purchasing groups for three reasons:

1. incentive to gain business;
2. fear of losing business; and
3. volume to be gained or lost.

When members dilute their participation in one group by giving partial support to others, the suppliers lose their motivation for acknowledging the central purchasing organization, and the effectiveness of the group's efforts is compromised.

Your hospital's participation in a group purchasing program increases your buying leverage and offers the expertise of another purchasing professional, the group director, to your staff. Not all groups will suit you and your hospital, and your selection of the right group is one of the important decisions you will make for your institution.

After you make your selection and join a group purchasing organization, your support for the group and its programs is essential to the success of the program. The agreements made are only as strong as the commitment of the individual members. It is far easier for a member to ruin a group purchasing program than to make it strong and successful. When purchasing or materiel managers are unable or unwilling to implement group contracts in their hospitals, or when these managers attempt to improve on selected group contracts to satisfy their egos, the performance of the group suffers. The right group for you and your hospital is the group to which you can give your wholehearted support.

Measuring savings from group purchasing

Dan B. Lang
Assistant Director
Halifax Hospital Medical Center
Daytona Beach, Florida

GROUP PURCHASING NETS TWO MILLION IN SAVINGS! reads a headline. Shared service hospital purchasing groups have indeed been reducing supply costs across the United States. However, current measurement methodologies may not be accurately computing the actual dollars saved.

This article presents a practical and realistic methodology for a hospital to calculate its group purchase savings. This method, the Standard Index Quantity Price Method (SIQP), estimates what a hospital would have been paying if it were not participating in a group.

CURRENT METHODOLOGIES

Calculating savings on a particular product during the first year of group purchase is a straightforward process. The difference between the prices a hospital pays before joining a group and those it pays afterwards are multiplied by the annual purchase volume. The result equals the amount of savings generated. Subsequent years' savings on the same product, however, are not as easy to compute since market prices fluctuate. The materiel manager will know each year's group purchase prices, of course, but has to estimate what the hospital *would* have been paying had it not been buying through a group.

Shared service groups in 15 states were contacted and asked to explain their methodologies for estimating savings on group purchases. Most groups computed first year savings in the manner just described. To calculate savings for subsequent years, however, the groups used widely varying methods.

Four groups applied the savings percentages from the initial contracts to gross group purchases of subsequent years. This percentage method may be accurate for the first year, but it unrealistically assumes that inflation rates in subsequent years will be the same for group and nongroup prices.

Two groups applied the annual increase in the Consumer Price Index (CPI) to pregroup prices to calculate what their hospitals would have been paying after the first year. Purchasing agents, however, through effective negotiations and competitive bidding, can keep their average price increases per item well below the CPI increase. In addition, different supply categories will have different inflation rates.

Another group extrapolated to all participating hospitals the savings percentage generated on initial contracts for new participants. Supply prices, however, vary so extensively among hospitals that ex-

trapolating one hospital's savings to another is inappropriate.

Other methods were used to estimate current market prices for purchases outside the group. In two cases, prices of nonparticipant hospitals were spot-checked to compute market averages. Again, this does not necessarily reflect the prices that each hospital can secure with effective purchasing practices. And inter-hospital price variance makes extrapolation from one hospital to another of dubious value.

One group counted the difference between manufacturer's list price and group price actually paid as its savings. Very few hospitals, however, actually pay full list prices. Another group called a meeting of participating purchasing agents and asked what they thought prices would be outside the group arrangement. This was a highly speculative method, particularly considering that these were agents who were paying group prices.

In one case, the difference between a contract's negotiated price increase cap and the manufacturer's general price increase was considered additional savings. Nongroup hospitals, however, are not restricted to one vendor and can seek alternate sources when a vendor's prices increase.

The final method of computing savings was simply to multiply gross purchases for all hospitals by an arbitrary factor, such as 10 percent.

In summary, the methods presently used by groups have a number of drawbacks and may not be accurately calculating savings. Inaccurate estimates of group purchase savings could lead to a number

> *Overstating savings could cause a group to be inappropriately satisfied with its current vendors and prices . . . an understatement of savings could cause hospitals to bypass group buying opportunities through which they could reduce costs.*

of problems. Overstating savings could cause a group to be inappropriately satisfied with its current vendors and prices and to continue buying products that are not adequately discounted. An understatement of savings could cause hospitals to bypass group buying opportunities through which they could in fact reduce costs.

SIQP METHOD

The SIQP Method computes hospital-specific inflation rates for each major category of supplies to predict what a particular hospital would have been paying for supplies outside the group. The categories correspond to the classifications already used by the hospital. Examples of supply categories are medical–surgical supplies, office supplies, dietary supplies, dietary food, linens, pharmaceuticals and house-keeping supplies.

These personalized inflation indices measure the purchasing performance of the hospital for each supply category. Efforts to reduce prices, achieve discounts and standardize products will be reflected in a low SIQP inflation index.

Annual supply costs can be affected by four factors:

- increase in overhead costs;
- increase in number of different types of items;
- increase in purchased quantity of each item; and
- increase in the price per item.

Therefore, purchasing effectiveness cannot be measured by total supply costs alone. The SIQP Method addresses the fourth factor, item price, by using two measures of price level increase: the standard index and the quantity price.

The supply sample

The materiel manager should review hospital inventories, identify the significant supply categories and select a reasonably representative sample of the highest dollar items in each category. In a recent review of the purchasing function of a 600-bed hospital, the sample consisted of all "A" items in an ABC inventory system. The 404 "A" items, which comprised 21 percent of the hospital's total 1,893 different inventory items, accounted for 80 percent of its total dollar volume of supplies. The study included nine major supply categories, with the medical-surgical category containing almost half of the total "A" items.

To measure price level changes, at least two years of data are required. If an item is substantially modified between years or not carried in both years, it should be omitted and the next highest dollar item selected to complete the sample. Since these sample items will form the basis for future analyses, only standard items should be included. There should be a reasonable expectation that the items will be used in future years. One-time purchases for unusual conditions should be excluded.

Measuring price level changes

Figure 1 displays the worksheet used to collect price data. The quantity price of an item is the most current invoice price, net of discounts, for the specific quantity usually purchased by the hospital. The quantity price for 4 × 4 dressings increased from $40.00 to $47.17, but the quantity purchased also changed. The 1981 price must be multiplied by the quantity conversion factor (1980 quantity divided by 1981 quantity) to yield a converted 1981 quantity price of $39.29. The standard index is computed by dividing this converted 1981 quantity price by the 1980 quantity price of $40.00 to yield .982.

At the bottom of Figure 1, the 1981 converted quantity price total for the medical–surgical category is divided by the 1980 quantity price total. This gives the standardized quantity price, which indicates a 3.7 percent annual price increase for medical–surgical supplies.

The summed standard index is divided by the number of items in the category to yield a 4.0 percent annual price increase.

The two indexes are needed to cover each other's weaknesses. Simply adding all the quantity prices may bias results since price changes in expensive items will outweigh price changes in inexpensive items. For example, a 25 percent increase in one $100 item is equivalent to a 25 percent increase in twenty $5 items. Since items also come in cases of varying size, their prices will be artificially weighted. A case of 1,000 will dominate over a case of

12. The quantity price index alone can thus be biased by varying prices and case sizes.

The summed standard index, when divided by the number of items, indicates the *average* percentage of price increase per item. This index is not influenced either by the number of items in a case or by the price of an item relative to other items.

Unfortunately, it would be inappropriate to use the standard index alone. If price savings were achieved on many low-dollar items while a few high-dollar items were allowed to inflate, the hospital could actually be paying more for its supplies while a deceptive decreasing average standard index would be reported, because more prices decreased than increased.

It is necessary to monitor both indexes. When they approximate each other, it is safer to draw conclusions about price change trends. As they diverge, it is necessary to examine the data sheets more closely to ascertain the causes of the variance.

Returning to the Figure 1 example, the two indexes may be averaged to yield a 1981 SIQP index of 1.0385, representing a 3.85 percent annual price increase for medical–surgical supplies. Preferable to the CPI for calculating what a hospital would probably be paying for its supplies outside the group contract, the SIQP index reflects the hospital's own purchasing performance in each supply category.

Group purchase savings

To calculate the savings produced by group buying, the materiel manager can

Item description [1]	Quantity				Quantity conversion factor	Quantity price			Standardized index
	Unit of measure June 1980 (2)	Case quantity June 1980 (3)	Unit of measure June 1981 (4)	Case quantity June 1981 (5)	(6) $(2 \times 3)/(4 \times 5)$	June 1980 (7)	June 1981 (8)	Quantity converted 1981 (9) $(6) \times (8)$	June 1981 (10) $(9)/(7)$
Steri-Pads, 4 × 4	100 box	25	100 box	30	.833	40.00	47.17	39.29	.982
Razor, Disp. Prep	50 case	1	100 case	1	.500	26.50	58.00	29.00	1.094
Exam Gloves, Disp.	25 box	24	25 box	24	1.000	104.00	108.50	108.50	1.043
Total						170.50		176.79	3.119

Standardized Quantity Price = 176.79/170.50 = 1.037
Average Standard Index = 3.119/3 = 1.040
SIQP Index = (1.037 + 1.040)/2 = 1.0385

Figure 1. Sample SIQP index calculation, medical–surgical supply category. *Only three items are listed for simplified illustration. This category will normally contain a much larger sample.

Item description* (1)	Pre-group price 1976	1977	1978	1979	1980	1981	SIQP converted pre-group price (2)	Group order quantity 1981 (3)	Quantity converted pre-group price (4) (3/1) × (2)	1981 group price (5)	Unit savings (6) (4) − (5)	Annual pur- chase volume (7)	Annual savings (8) (6) × (7)
SIQP indexes	1.099	1.076	1.066	1.061	1.050	1.0385							
Tape, adhesive 2″, 6 can		4.50					4.91	6 can	4.91	4.25	0.66	3,500	2,310
Bandaid, plastic 1 × 3, 100 box.			1.50				1.74	50 box	0.87	0.70	0.17	6,000	1,020
Blade, surgical #10, 144 box					25.00		25.96	144 box	25.96	22.92	3.04	200	608
Mask, OR, 300 case						42.00	42.00	250 case	35.00	33.00	2.00	1,000	2,000
Total savings (medical–surgical category)													5,938

Figure 2. Sample calculation of group purchase savings, medical–surgical supply category. *These items are different from the ones in Figure 1. When analyzing group purchase savings, the SIQP index calculations of Figure 1 should not include the group purchased items. Their inclusion could reduce the SIQP index, thus understating group purchase savings.

use a worksheet like the one in Figure 2 for each supply category. Each supply item currently group purchased is entered into the worksheet along with the current group purchase price, the pregroup purchase price in the year of initial contract and the current annual purchase volume.

The SIQP indexes for this supply category are entered for each year across the top of the worksheet. The pregroup price is multiplied by the SIQP index for each subsequent year to derive the SIQP converted pregroup price for 1981. The pregroup price must also be quantity converted to be comparable to today's price. The 1981 group price is then subtracted from this quantity converted pregroup price to yield the unit saving. Finally, the unit saving is multiplied by annual purchase volume to derive the total savings generated on this item.

Three procedures should be followed when using the SIQP index. First, when analyzing group purchase savings, the SIQP index calculation should be based on items *not* being group purchased. Group purchased items could bring the total SIQP index down, thus lowering the estimate of savings. Separate SIQP analyses can be performed for group and nongroup prices and easily consolidated to measure overall purchasing performance.

Second, pregroup prices for some items may not be found in the records if the initial contracts were signed many years earlier. In these cases, the materiel manager should estimate a price that could be obtained based on what is current outside the group. In fact, the materiel manager may occasionally be able to accurately estimate the market prices of current items, either from recent vendor offers or from a current vendor price list showing a lower price than the SIQP estimated price. In those instances, the materiel manager's estimate should be entered instead of the SIQP estimate in column 2 of Figure 2.

Finally, the Figure 1 worksheet may be extended to include multiple years of data. The materiel manager may be pleasantly surprised to discover that during the last few years he or she has actually contained supply cost increases below the CPI.

Introducing SIQP

Group purchasing organizations do not and should not have the extra time and staff to perform these calculations for all member hospitals. The group could, however, prepare and distribute SIQP worksheets, establish criteria for hospitals to follow and train the hospital members to evaluate savings under group purchasing. Within three to four weeks, the hospitals could perform the calculations and report their savings to the group, which could sum them to get the total savings for the group.

The group may provide benefits other than purchase price savings. Product standardization, improved vendor services and reductions in local market prices for nonmember hospitals are possible positive effects resulting from the activities of a purchasing group.

The SIQP Method measures purchase price levels only. Under group arrangements, additional savings may be generated from reductions in inventory carrying costs, number of purchase orders or overhead costs. If these savings can be systematically measured, they should be added to the savings from purchase price reductions.

The SIQP Method is an excellent tool for monitoring category-specific price levels of hospital supplies. The SIQP index is useful not only for measuring purchasing effectiveness and group purchasing savings, but also for assessing prime vendor prices, evaluating contracts with price increase caps and forecasting future supply prices based on past performance.

When group purchase savings are esti-

The SIQP index is useful not only for measuring group purchasing savings, but also for assessing prime vendor prices, evaluating contracts with price increase caps and forecasting future supply prices.

mated under the SIQP Method, a higher level of credibility will be assigned to the newspaper headlines that extol huge savings.

Group purchasing makes sense: an administrator's perspective

Richard L. Sims
Administrator
Doctors Hospital
Columbus, Ohio

HOSPITAL ADMINISTRATORS are faced daily with pressures stemming from the financial environment; health care delivery needs and expectations of the consuming public; technology changes; shortage of key personnel; and governmental regulations and restraints. In particular, hospital costs continue to rise and so do pressures to contain them.

The growing concern of government, and of business, labor and consumer groups as well, is that hospitals may soon price themselves out of reach of the economy's ability to pay for health care. With the new administration promising tax cuts and reductions in federal programs, health care costs will again be under close scrutiny. Tightening the screws on Medicare-Medicaid and other third party reimbursement plans may be the only way for the Reagan Administration to get a handle on rising health care costs.

In this setting, hospitals and their administrators must view cost effectiveness as a key element in achieving their goals—unless they are ready for more regulation, more controls and more take-over of management. A very useful strategy for cost containment is group purchasing.

THE DEVELOPMENT OF GROUP PURCHASING

The group purchasing concept is not new, although it has become more popular in recent years. What is probably the best known and most successful attempt to contain the cost of supplies and equipment began in the early 1950s with the Hospital Bureau of New York. Hospital membership was voluntary and accompanied by a fee. For the first time in the United States, member hospitals were able to participate in purchasing contracts through the Bureau.

Hospitals over the years have become more and more interested in this approach to cost containment. Religious orders that own and operate a group of hospitals, for example, have consolidated their individual efforts by negotiating purchasing contracts for the entire group. The Third Order of St. Francis in Peoria, Illinois, performed this function for its hospitals for several years and then expanded its field of activities to allow nonaffiliated institutions to become members.

Many metropolitan hospital councils have put together excellent group purchasing programs for their members in the interest of cost savings through joint efforts. Even the for-profit sector of the hospital industry has purchasing contracts as a branch of consulting and management activities. And, logically, hospitals in a

given geographic area often unite in a local or state organization in an attempt to obtain the best buy for their dollars. The balance of this article examines the experience of one such local hospital purchasing group.

THE COLUMBUS EXPERIENCE

Hospital administrators in Columbus, Ohio, through the Mid-Ohio Health Planning Federation, initiated local group purchasing in 1971. Ten Columbus hospitals joined together to form an area hospital purchasing program. Early targets included a common elevator maintenance contract and several shared services: laundry, medical laboratory, data processing and collection of accounts receivable. A Purchasing Advisory Committee was appointed in January 1974, and a statement of purpose and operating guidelines was prepared.

The program's goals and procedures

The essential narrative of this document was and remains as follows:

The purpose of this purchasing program is to provide for the nonprofit hospitals in the area the advantage of cooperating in the purchasing of products and services, thereby benefiting the economic and efficient operation of those hospitals.

Subject to the approval of the participating hospitals, the Franklin County Administrators Council will supervise and direct the purchasing program. The Administrators Council shall negotiate purchasing programs on behalf of the participating hospitals for their approval.

The Administrators Council will designate a

Purchasing Advisory Committee with a purchasing representative from each participating hospital.

The Administrators Council will select items for group purchasing based upon the recommendation of the Purchasing Advisory Committee.

The bid proposals will be analyzed by the Purchasing Advisory Committee and their recommendations, together with the bid proposals, will be submitted to the Administrators Council for review.[1]

A formal procedure was adopted for purchasing selected products. It involved the systematic selection and study of products by the Purchasing Advisory Committee, solicitation of proposals from vendors, analysis of proposals and final selection of product or service. (See boxed material.)

Program results

The Columbus group purchasing program achieved moderate success, as evidenced by the approximately 12 percent annual savings. Table 1 shows some typical savings, as well as level of hospital participation.

In 1978 the Columbus hospital purchasing effort split off from the Mid-Ohio Health Planning Federation for two reasons: The project was becoming too time consuming for the limited federation staff available for it, and a change in the Health Planning law made it undesirable for a health systems agency to operate a shared service program for a "provider" group. The ten Columbus hospitals formed Hospital Shared Services, Inc.

Purchasing Advisory Committee: Procedural Outline

Procedure	Primary responsibility
Select potential product based on established criteria and appoint a project coordinator	Purchasing Advisory Committee
Conduct survey for participation at Purchasing Advisory Committee meeting	Purchasing Advisory Committee
Prepare survey for potential product item	Purchasing Advisory Committee
Prepare results of survey	Federation Staff
Report results of survey to Purchasing Advisory Committee	Federation Staff
Select vendors	Purchasing Advisory Committee
Using survey results, prepare and send out proposal requests to vendors	Federation Staff, Purchasing Advisory Committee, Project Committee
Open proposals	Federation Staff
Prepare proposal analysis and report to Purchasing Advisory Committee	Federation Staff
Select best proposal	Purchasing Advisory Committee
Report recommendations to Administrators Council	Administrative Representative
Invite hospitals to participate in program on voluntary basis	Purchasing Advisory Committee, Administrators Council, Federation Staff

(HSSI), a nonprofit 501C-6 organization for the purpose of expanding their group purchasing activities. HSSI results are impressive, and cost savings continue to far outweigh the cost of establishing the organization.

The shift to larger associations

The quantity and quality (of products and contracts) of HSSI group purchasing increased through 1979. National organizations, however, were making inroads into Central Ohio. One large Columbus area hospital joined the Volunteer Hospitals of America and another elected to go with a prime supplier. This turn of events caused the rest of the local hospitals to reconsider their own position with regard to local vs. much larger associations able to obtain higher discounts on contracts. The result

was a decrease in local group purchasing activities during 1980.

Three Columbus hospitals have since joined a large purchasing corporation representing over 100 hospitals throughout the country. Thus the local effort has substantially diminished. However, the shift to larger associations promises even greater cost containment than originally envisioned in 1974.

Whether a hospital joins a local or national purchasing group, the administrator must be willing to:

1. commit total support to the group;
2. be flexible with regard to specifications and standardization, and encourage staff physicians and others to accept equivalent products; and
3. block efforts of vendors to undercut the bidding process.

Table 1. Columbus Area Hospital Purchasing Program: typical savings and participation

Project	1979 current dollar volume	Demonstrated savings 1979	No. of participating hospitals
Dairy products	$ 350,396	$ 33,060	8
Paper products	220,876	46,781	8
Lighting supplies	30,148	11,000	9
X-ray film	859,365	40,826	6
Stationery supplies	76,147	24,830	9
Sutures	308,011	8,273	5
Bread	87,579	19,744	9
Shoe covers	18,197	11,454	6
Underpads	42,655	13,578	3
Monitoring chart paper	14,196	4,943	6
Ampicillin	50,772	5,783	4
Thermometers	56,711	24,199	7
Linen	86,887	10,628	6
Duplicating paper	88,212	18,495	8
Seven Up	40,000	5,000	9
		negotiated disc.	
Total	$2,330,152	$278,594	

Source: Hospital Shared Services, Inc.

Another shift in the direction of the Columbus Group Purchasing Program took place in 1983 when the group decided to broaden the organization from local to regional. In Central Ohio forty hospitals found it expedient to join together in a new trade association—Hospital Association of Central Ohio (HACO).

The group purchasing programs of HSSI were folded into the new HACO and members can choose to participate in services on a cafeteria-style basis. It is yet to be demonstrated how the expansion of the program from ten to forty hospitals, and one county to a regional multi-county system will work. It is anticipated, however, that many more hospitals will take advantage of cost-saving opportunities.

Above all, commitment is the key, and the overriding concern must be to maximize cost containment in the purchase of goods and services. In Columbus and other cities, hospitals have just begun to scratch the surface and develop the real potential of group purchasing and shared services.

PROBLEMS IN ESTABLISHING GROUP PURCHASING

Once a hospital's chief executive officer has anointed the project and announced management's support for group purchasing, the task of implementing the commitment falls to the materiel manager or purchasing director. And it is not always an easy task.

Traditional relationships upset

The chief purchasing officer in any organization, if he or she has been on board for a considerable time, has developed friendship and loyalty with detail people, manufacturers' agents and local suppliers. These individuals have been helpful to the hospital in getting supplies in time of shortage, leaking warnings of industry-planned price increases, providing rush service favors to eliminate supply outage crises, and informing staff and departments of product improvement and technological changes. In addition, some sales representatives cultivate the favor of hospital purchasing agents through gifts and other amenities. The administrator and top executive managers can also be subject to these same enticements.

Group purchasing endangers this traditional system. The sales representatives, who after all are lobbyists for their products, fear the diminished product choice and decision-making ability at the individual hospital level. They in turn put fear in the minds of hospital purchasers that this new group action will break up the close, friendly relationships which have previously worked to the advantage of the hospital and its agent. Worse yet, salespeople and suppliers have been known to unite against the group bidding process and either boycott it or work together to maintain current prices thus eliminating competitive bidding.

Local opposition

Powerful local firms may perceive group purchasing as a threat to their share of the competitive market. Such firms may argue that group purchasing will threaten the area's free market. Many hospitals solicit charitable contributions to their foundations or development funds from local and national firms. Group purchasing tends to dry up these sources of gifts, particularly when a firm has recently lost the hospital's business to group purchasing.

The "sour grapes" response to the introduction of group purchasing must be endured for a short period while the system demonstrates its advantages. Once its cost savings *and* its impartiality are demonstrated, vendors' fears allayed and the story told to the community, the temporary bad public relations turn positive.

Turning bad public relations into good

Business and industry groups, which have used basically the same type of joint programs for decades, become the strong supporters of group purchasing efforts by hospitals as do Blue Cross and other payers. Their collective commendation may include a gentle barb that: "It's about time hospitals started working together for the good of containing rising health care costs." They view group purchasing as one

bright light at the end of a tunnel of bad news on ever-rising hospital rates.

In turn, many of these same industry and community leaders become advocates of the Voluntary Effort (VE) and, if asked, are pleased to be helpful to local or state VE programs.

Thus group purchasing and shared services are not only economically beneficial, they also boost hospital-community relations by proving to the public that the hospital is acting effectively and in the best interest of patients.

To make group purchasing work, however, requires the best efforts of top hospital executives and materiel managers to initiate and implement each hospital's involvement. It also takes leadership to gain the dedication of others to the cause so that a total united group effort can be successful. Finally, it takes courage for the group to withstand the criticism that is bound to surface when so big a change is made in traditional purchasing relationships. The rewards to both the individual hospital and the health care industry, however, are well worth the risks and the efforts.

REFERENCE

1. Administrators' Council of the Mid-Ohio Health Planning Federation, Columbus, Ohio. Minutes of Meeting, January 1974.

Evaluation of group purchasing programs: a proposed methodology

Donald J. Siegle
Vice President
Hospital Council of Western Pennsylvania
Pittsburgh, Pennsylvania

GROUP PURCHASING programs became successful so rapidly in the 1970s that there was hardly time to evaluate the elements of their success. Since very few programs were the result of written plans, it was difficult to measure the deviation from plan, which is usually the basis of evaluation. However, if group purchasing is going to continue to prosper in the years ahead, each program should begin to look carefully at its results in terms not only of *what* happened, but of *why* it happened.

Systematic program evaluation can provide an in-depth analysis of the elements of a program and its procedures. Schaefer, in his book on program evaluation in health planning, makes it clear that any major administrative function that involves decision making should include evaluation.[1] He maintains that although much evaluation takes place in intuitive, sporadic, informal and unregularized ways, it is desirable that evaluation be systematic.

However, a systematic evaluation can also be so complex and cover so many subjects that its results become unwieldy. The goal is a methodology that is simple and useful. Such an approach is offered here.

The fundamental act in the evaluation process is *comparison* of program elements or results against *norms* or desired states. Norms are made operational through the use of *criteria* or measurable components of a norm used to reflect a desired state. As an example, if a group negotiated a price on an item, it might choose to measure it against the criterion of the top 10 percent of prices paid by other groups. If the group's price meets the criterion, it may not be necessary to make changes in future negotiation methods for that product. The desired state is not perfection, or the lowest price in the world, but rather a level of satisfaction.

Since evaluators must deal with assessing relative worth and comparative effectiveness, measurable answers to questions are important. If the question asked is whether a given price negotiation results in savings, a simple answer of yes does not permit systematic evaluation. It is necessary to be a great deal more specific in quantitative terms about the savings *and* to compare them with specific criteria.

The proposed methodology offers a set of yes/no questions relating to various aspects of group purchasing: policy manuals; performance of the staff; the effect on prices; vendor potential and performance; the survey of market conditions; the deci-

sion-making process; and the byproducts of group purchasing. Each question relates to a criterion of satisfaction, and the answers to each can be rated in points from zero to ten, with seven points or 70 percent being the satisfaction level or norm. This level can of course be set at any value by the evaluator. Each answer that falls below the norm should include a comment by the evaluator, consisting of constructive criticism and positive recommendation.

THE POLICY MANUAL

The availability of a written purchasing policy manual has come to be recognized as one hallmark of a mature, competent and professional purchasing organization.[2] Without clear policy statements to implement policies, the ability of the purchasing organization to communicate not only with its management and the diversified areas it serves, but within every phase of the purchasing operation is severely limited.[3] If the policy manual is written clearly, the entire purchasing process will move smoothly and proceed as planned. An evaluation of policy manuals might include the following questions, all formatted like question 1 for yes/no answers and the zero-to-ten points ratings already described:

1. Is there a written policy and procedure manual? _____ Yes _____ No _____ Points
2. Does the manual clearly define the purchasing process step by step?
3. Was the policy manual approved by management? committee members? legal advisor? financial auditor?

4. Is the policy manual reviewed and revised at least every three years?

PERFORMANCE OF THE STAFF

Management uses staff evaluation to become fully aware of the activities of each department, to share in the solution of its problems and to measure the effectiveness of the people managing the department.[4] To properly evaluate the purchasing function, it is necessary to consider carefully the climate in which it is

---

To properly evaluate the purchasing function, it is necessary to consider carefully the climate in which it is operating.

---

operating. The evaluator must make every effort to eliminate human bias and discrimination when evaluating staff. Evaluators can apply the following questions, all formatted like question 1, in evaluating purchasing program staff:

1. Do the members feel the staff are competent, friendly and interested in their problems? (Contact a sample of member hospital personnel by phone.) ____Yes ____No ____Points
2. Are the communication documents clearly written? (Letters, invitations to bid, contracts, surveys, minutes, etc.)
3. Are contract notices sent to hospitals, and are they clear and informative? (Do they contain price and other order placement information?)
4. Are reports and records accurate and complete? (Survey analyses, annual report, bid analyses)
5. Does the organization enjoy financial stability?
6. Do the staff work well with vendors? (Contact a sample of vendors by phone.)
7. Do the staff attend continuing education programs and stay active with local purchasing associations?
8. Do the staff show initiative on the job? (New projects each year.)
9. Have the staff used research to assist in decision making? (Laboratory tests, written reports, product evaluations, value analysis, etc.)
10. Do reports to management include results of contract negotiations, status of objectives and major conditions affecting the program?
11. Is the program managed at a cost comparable to those of other programs of similar size and age? Note: The average purchasing program has 79 member hospitals with a total of 14,860 beds, is 14 years old, has annual participation of $44 million, average participation of $246 per bed per month and operates at a cost of 0.7 percent of total dollar hospital participation.[5]
12. Do the staff publish a newsletter or participate regularly in a corporate newsletter?
13. Do the staff visit hospitals or have a traveling representative?
14. Are committee members given orientation programs and objectives each year?

EFFECT ON PRICES

One of the easiest ways to secure lower prices is to consolidate quantities. This is the basic reason why centralized purchasing was established.[6] The very existence of a group purchasing program changes the relationship between supply and demand[7] and can affect prices in many ways. Evaluation questions should look at whether the purchasing program utilizes the following methods to effect lower prices:

1. Quantity consolidation resulting in lower vendor cost per unit?[8]

   ____ Yes ____ No ____ Points

2. Quality standardization resulting in inventory reduction?

3. Negotiation techniques using teams of volunteer hospital personnel?

4. Price stability and longer firm price periods?

5. Reduced freight costs due to quantity consolidation?

6. Better cash terms due to guarantees of groups?

7. Competition from increased number of interested vendors?

8. Contract commitment enabling vendors to plan better?

9. Escalation control, using wholesale market reports?

10. Warehousing, dealing directly with producers and manufacturers and providing distribution?[9]

In addition, other useful questions might be:

11. Does the program document net price trends over multiyear periods?

12. Does the program calculate the dollar savings on each contract, total and by hospital?

13. Does the program group products into logical packages that may be competitively bid by many vendors yet be more enticing than individual products? (Example: "total electrical maintenance products" rather than merely "electric bulbs.")

VENDOR POTENTIAL AND PERFORMANCE

Group purchasing programs have the same problems as other procurement agents in selecting the right vendor. However, using peer groups to maintain a bidder's list generally will produce a wider variety of potential vendors. Groups have a tendency to reach out further to stimulate competition. Some groups visit vendors and prepare reports on vendor potential. In addition, vendor evaluation reports may be prepared after a period of experience with certain vendors. It is also possible to devise a vendor complaint system that attempts to deal with problems as they come up. Questions for evaluating how a group deals with vendors are:

1. Does the group maintain a bidder's list for each contract? ____ Yes ____ No ____ Points

2. Is there a policy for adding and deleting vendors on the bidder's list?

3. Is there a system for recording and assessing the performance of vendors?

4. Is that system of judging performance used as a reference when the next contract with a vendor is negotiated?[10]

THE SURVEY OF MARKET CONDITIONS

The evaluation of a purchasing program is meaningless without a market survey—

> *The evaluation of a purchasing program is meaningless without an array of data and information that portrays the conditions existing before the program was implemented.*

an array of data and information that portrays the conditions existing before the program was implemented.[11] Such a survey generally requests information on what each hospital is presently purchasing and what the hospital expects the group purchasing program to provide.

However, the attitude of member hospital personnel may be a serious barrier to the collection of such data.[12] Since the survey of market conditions is usually on a voluntary basis, the hospital cooperation may depend upon the commitment of hospital management to cost containment, the background and education of the hospital personnel and the availability of data.

Most groups, when surveying market conditions prior to contract negotiation, regard their survey as representative of the group if it includes hospitals of various sizes and services, and teaching affiliations. Also, groups consider their survey participation as successful if they get replies from 40 percent of their members. The Direct Mail Association also feels that groups of associated members should receive a survey return of 30 to 40 percent.[13] The survey may be the backbone of the program. It should elicit specific data about product size, strength, weight, package, quantity, quality, service and price. In evaluating a group purchasing program's survey, the following questions are useful:

1. Was the initial market survey returned by at least 40 percent of the potential participants? ____ Yes ____ No ____ Points
2. Did the survey include a random sample of hospitals by size, services, teaching status and geography?
3. Did the survey determine the quantity and quality of materials being purchased prior to the introduction of group purchasing?
4. Was a survey analysis report compiled and sent to hospital members?
5. Is there a market survey for every new contract negotiated?
6. Does the survey include the price of every item purchased within the product grouping?
7. Does the survey include the name of the vendors being utilized?
8. Is the average price per unit calculated in such a way that it may be compared to national data available?

THE DECISION-MAKING PROCESS

The group purchasing organization is faced with the serious work of deciding which products to bid, which vendors to approve and which vendor deserves the contract. If the group's policies are well written and well understood by its committees, the process of decision making is quite clear. If a group is to act as "one" and make a decision which satisfies the majority, some of its members must compromise and possibly give up their individual objectives. However, since technical expertise is much greater added together than isolated, the group's decisions will be based upon optimal criteria.[14]

Group decision making may take a little longer and be subject to a greater variety of interpretations, but if the majority is satisfied, there is real strength in the final product.

The use of subcommittees allows most groundwork for decisions to be completed by a number of small, manageable groups. This decentralization allows the program to work concurrently on many different contracts. The group purchasing staff meets with subcommittees to act as a catalyst and to provide them with necessary product samples, laboratory reports, etc. The subcommittee works with these data and then makes a recommendation to the full committee.

The evaluation of a group purchasing program's decision-making process may include the following questions:

1. Are the committees and subcommittees given sufficient specific information to properly make their decisions on the award of the contract?
   a. Are bids systematically compared?
      ____ Yes ____ No ____ Points
   b. Are results compared to the survey information prior to decision making?
   c. Are prices listed in comparison format?
   d. Do the bids include all sizes and types of products?
   e. Does bid analysis make note of which items have heavy usage?
   f. Does the bid analysis include factors other than price, such as freight, firm pricing, minimum orders, cash discounts and sales service?
2. Is there a democratic process of arriving at the final decision/recommendations with a motion made by the

subcommittee and discussion by the full committee?
3. Is there a count made of the membership's vote in order to show the committee the group opinion?
4. Is the decision-making process explained in the policy manual?

THE BYPRODUCTS OF GROUP PURCHASING

The average group purchasing program is about fourteen years old and is kept quite busy providing contract administration. However, as the number of contracts increases and participation by hospitals mounts, each purchasing program should be given funds to establish byproduct programs.

Although price control is a major program objective, a purchasing program can also play an important role in assisting hospitals to meet other goals. The staff of the program should meet with hospital personnel and study the problems of the purchasing department. Since many purchasing departments have small staffs, many of their research and education planning needs can better be met through the group, taking advantage of group dynamics and the economics of large numbers.

If there is no local purchasing society, the purchasing program staff can assist in

As the number of its contracts increases and participation by hospitals mounts, each purchasing program should be given funds to establish byproduct programs in areas such as research and continuing education.

organizing a chapter of a national association. The experience gained by members in organizing and managing such a chapter is a form of management training. The group purchasing staff can also assist in developing continuing education programs that will interest all members, regardless of their educational backgrounds.

In addition to education, the group purchasing staff can assist hospitals in developing modern systems such as materiel management. This is such a major program that many hospitals may not be able to plan and implement it without consulting outside experts. Group purchasing staff can assist hospitals in obtaining this consultation and keeping the costs reasonable.

Purchasing staff in hospitals are kept so busy carrying out their daily tasks that they are seldom able to conduct the research that they see is necessary. The group purchasing program can put into effect sophisticated research techniques, such as Value Analysis, on behalf of its members.

In the course of these byproduct programs, the program staff can take pride in seeing members of the purchasing group grow more capable and more united in spirit. The results will be quite noticeable by hospital management.

It may seem unfair to evaluate a group purchasing program along these lines, but where this progress into byproduct programs is necessary for future stability, evaluation questions would be:

1. Does the program sponsor continuing education and assist, or help develop, the local purchasing association? _____ Yes _____ No _____ Points
2. Do the program staff assist member hospitals in implementing materiel management programs?
3. Does the program provide product and function research, such as Value Analysis?
4. Does the program provide price review audits or other internal audits to its members?
5. Are there any other byproduct programs?

If occasional physical examinations are good practice in keeping individuals healthy, then is it not a good idea to keep group purchasing programs healthy through periodic self-evaluations? The proposed self-evaluation described here is quite subjective, but if seriously applied, will clearly point out areas for program improvement. There are 60 questions. The highest potential score is 600 points. With the satisfaction level set at 70 percent, a minimum of 420 points would be required for a purchasing program to be judged satisfactory. However, evaluators should be encouraged to write recommendations for every question whose ratings indicate improvement is needed. By closing the gaps between norms and actuality, group purchasing programs can strengthen their position and thereby merit more serious consideration by members and vendors.

REFERENCES

1. Schaefer, M. *Evaluation and Decision-Making in Health Planning* (Chapel Hill: University of North Carolina 1973).

2. McAleer, J.A. *NAPM Purchasing Guide* (New York: National Association of Purchasing Managers 1968).

3. Aljian, G., ed. *Purchasing Handbook* (New York:

McGraw-Hill 1973).

4. Wada, H. *Purchasing Handbook*, Aljian, G., ed.

5. "Annual Statistical Review." Paper presented to Group Purchasing Group at annual meeting, New Orleans, October 1982.

6. Aljian. *Purchasing Handbook.*

7. Ammer, D. *Hospital Materials Management* (Boston: Northeastern University 1973).

8. Aljian. *Purchasing Handbook.*

9. Ammer. *Hospital Materials Management.*

10. Hospital Council of Western Pennsylvania. *Group Purchasing Policy Manual* 3rd ed. (Warrendale, Pa.: HCWP 1971) p. 18, Section I3.

11. Schaefer. *Evaluation and Decision-Making in Health Planning.*

12. Ohio State University, School of Business. *A Survey of Attitudes and Hospital Group Purchasing* (Columbus, Ohio: OSU 1972).

13. Schaefer. *Evaluation and Decison-Making in Health Planning.*

14. Napier, R.W. and Gershenfeld, M.K. *Groups: Theory and Experience* (Boston: Houghton Mifflin Co. 1973).

Index

W

Z